Emergency Orthopaedic Radiology

Emergency Orthopaedic Radiology

Robert J. Neviaser, M.D.
Professor
Department of Orthopaedic Surgery
School of Medicine and Health Sciences
George Washington University
Washington, D.C.

Larry S. Eisenfeld, M.D.
Orthopedic Associates
Fort Myers, Florida

Sam W. Wiesel, M.D.
Professor
Department of Orthopaedic Surgery
School of Medicine and Health Sciences
George Washington University
Washington, D.C.

Randall J. Lewis, M.D.
Associate Clinical Professor
Department of Orthopaedic Surgery
School of Medicine and Health Sciences
George Washington University
Washington, D.C.

CHURCHILL LIVINGSTONE
New York, Edinburgh, London, and Melbourne 1985

Production editor: Charlie Lebeda
Production supervisor: Kerry A. O'Rourke
Compositor: Progressive Typographers, Inc.
Printer/Binder: Halliday Lithograph

Distributed in the United Kingdom by Churchill Livingstone, Robert Stevenson House, 1-3 Baxter's Place, Leith Walk, Edinburgh EH1 3AF and by associated companies, branches and representatives throughout the world.

First published 1985

Printed in U.S.A.

ISBN 0-443-08188-3

7 6 5 4 3 2 1

Library of Congress Cataloging in Publication Data

Main entry under title:

Emergency orthopaedic radiology.

Includes bibliographies and index.
1. Spine — Radiography. 2. Spine — Wounds and injuries — Diagnosis. 3. Extremities (Anatomy) — Radiography. 4. Extremities (Anatomy) — Wounds and injuries — Diagnosis. I. Neviaser, Robert J. [DNLM: 1. Spine — radiography. 2. Extremities — radiography. 3. Emergencies. WE 725 E53]
RD533.E46 1985 617'.3707'57 84-23679
ISBN 0-443-08188-3

Dedicated to John Pletch Adams, M.D.,
for his guidance and support

Preface

This book is intended to assist the physician treating a person with an injury to the spine or extremities. That physician may be a family practitioner, emergency room physician, or even an orthopaedic surgeon. Although there are a number of texts on emergency medicine and radiology, they do not contain much material on orthopaedic injuries. This is unfortunate since injuries to the spine and extremities are among those most commonly seen in any emergency room or out-patient setting. As a result, we have included normal radiographs as well as those illustrating fractures and dislocations. We have accompanied them in specific instances with line drawings to make the interpretation of the radiographs easier.

The text is divided on the basis of regional anatomy. This should facilitate the location of any injury by anatomic area. The format of the respective chapters includes a brief discussion of the mechanism of injury, the clinical representation, the radiographic findings, associated injuries, and potential complications. Emergency treatment is suggested. It is hoped that this will aid the treating physician in making an accurate diagnosis instituting appropriate initial therapy.

The goal of this book is to improve the care of the patient in the emergency setting. It hopefully will enhance the relationship between the initial treating physician and the orthopaedic surgeon who will follow the patient subsequently.

It is appropriate to express our appreciation to those who have contributed with their time and efforts so generously to help us complete this work. James Kendrick of the Audio Visual Department of the George Washington University School of Medicine has been invaluable in the reproduction of the illustrations. The Departments of Radiology of both the George Washington University Hospital and the Washington Hospital Center have been generous in allowing us to use their teaching files. The art work was done by Ann Bignell with highly professional skill. The manuscript revisions have been undertaken with grace by Terry Place, Saundra Long, Gloria Wilson, Maureen Church, Renee Younger, Gayla Smith, and Sue Turner.

Contents

1. Fracture Terminology 1

PART I THE SPINE

2. The Cervical Spine 11
3. The Thoracolumbar Spine 35

PART II THE UPPER EXTREMITIES

4. The Shoulder and Humerus 57
5. The Elbow 83
6. The Forearm 101
7. The Wrist 113
8. The Hand 139

PART III THE LOWER EXTREMITIES

9. The Pelvis 173
10. The Hip and Femur 185
11. The Knee 211
12. The Tibia and Fibula 231
13. The Ankle 237
14. The Foot 257

Index 275

Emergency Orthopaedic Radiology

1 Fracture Terminology

The various terms used in this book are commonly employed in orthopedics. In order to establish a satisfactory means of communication between the examining physician and his consultant, the following definitions will be helpful.

1. *Open fracture* (Fig. 1-1). A fracture in which there is communication between the external environment and the fracture site.
2. *Closed fracture.* A fracture in which the skin is intact and there is no communication with the environment.

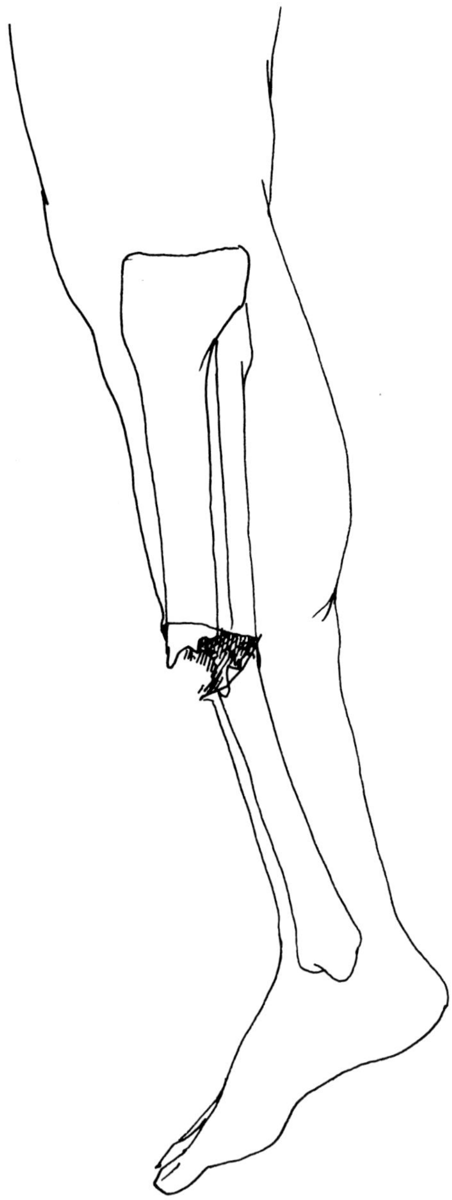

Fig. 1-1. Open fracture.

3. *Comminuted fracture* (Fig. 1-2). Three or more fracture fragments are present.
4. *Transverse fracture* (Fig. 1-3). The fracture line is perpendicular or nearly so to the longitudinal axis of the bone. It is usually a result of direct trauma.

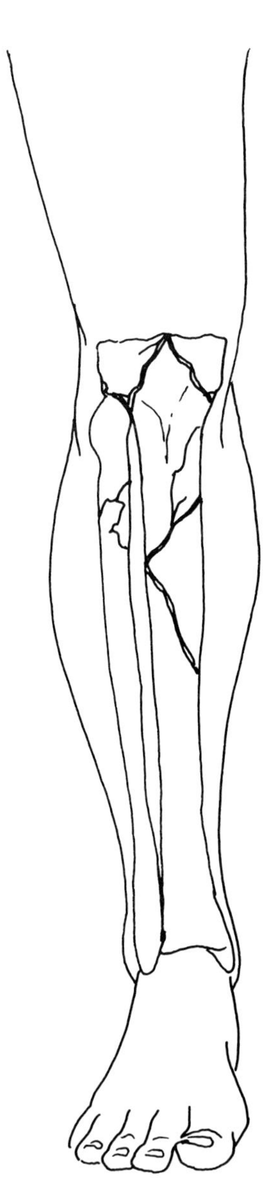

Fig. 1-2. Closed fracture.

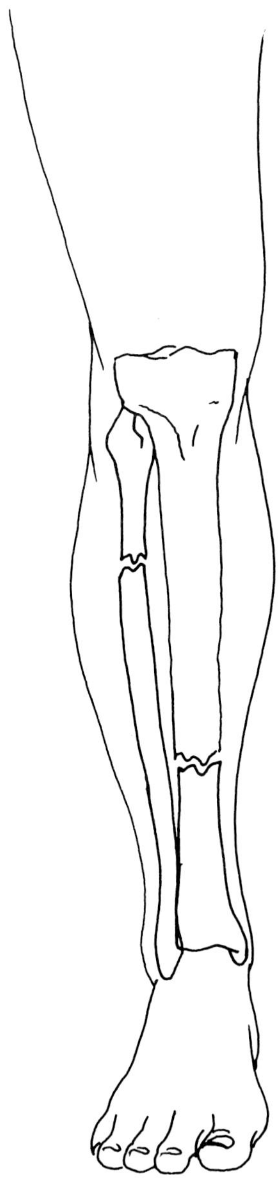

Fig. 1-3. Transverse fracture.

5. *Oblique/spiral fracture* (Fig. 1-4). The fracture line is usually at an angle of 45 degrees to the transverse or longitudinal axis of the bone. It is the result of an indirect or twisting force.
6. *Stellate fracture.* As implied, the fracture is in a starshaped configuration with fracture lines radiating from a central point. It is usually the result of a severe, direct trauma.

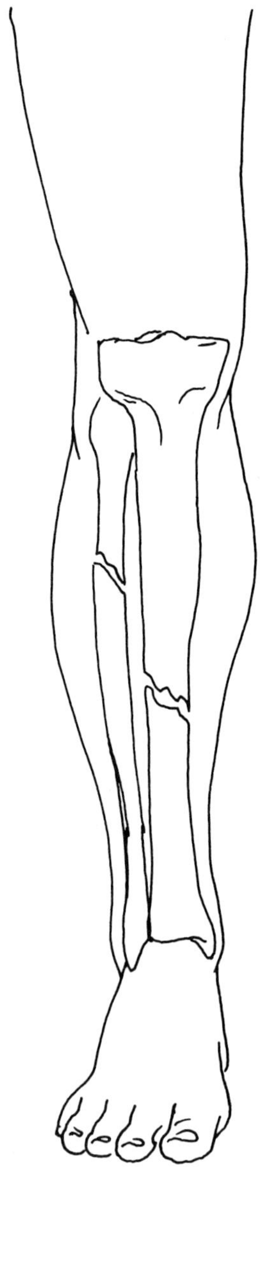

Fig. 1-4. Oblique/spiral fracture.

7. *Avulsion fracture.* A fragment of bone of varying size has been avulsed with insertion of a ligament or a tendon.
8. *Subluxation.* Imperfect alignment of the opposing sides of a joint. There is still some contact between the articular surfaces of the respective sides of the joint, but the alignment is abnormal.
9. *Dislocation.* The opposing sides of any joint are no longer in contact at all.
10. *Varus alignment* (Fig. 1-5). The alignment of the distal limb of a fracture or a joint that deviates toward a midline.

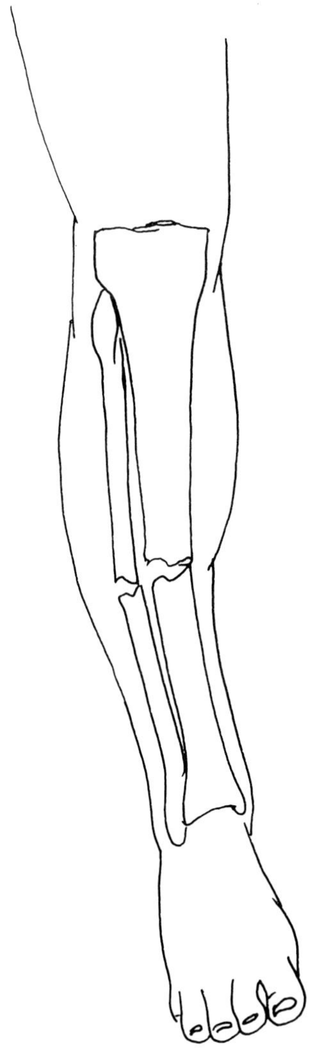

Fig. 1-5. Varus alignment.

11. *Valgus alignment* (Fig. 1-6). A distal limb of a fracture or joint that deviates away from midline.

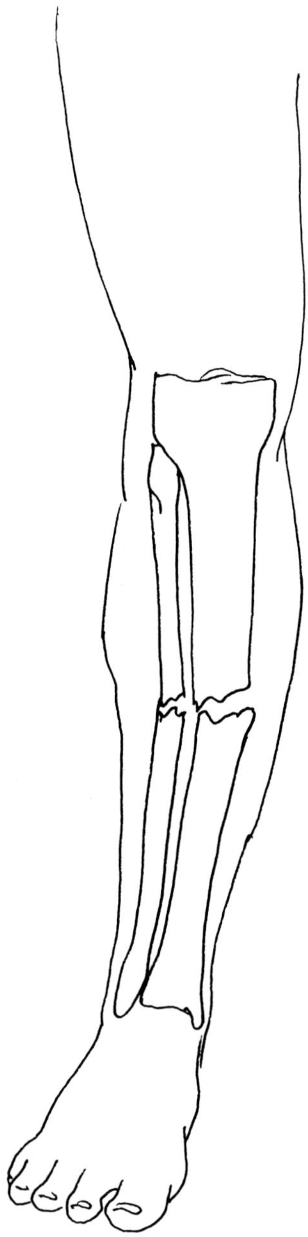

Fig. 1-6. Valgus alignment.

12. *Displacement* (Fig. 1-7). Abnormal alignment of fracture fragments either in the longitudinal or transverse plane.
13. *Angulation* (Fig. 1-8). The tilting of a distal limb or fragment of a fracture creating an angle at the site of injury.

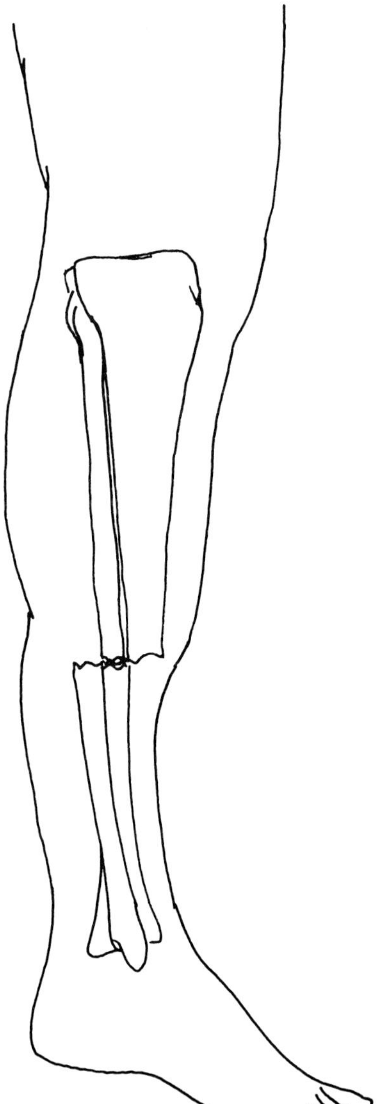

Fig. 1-7. Displacement.

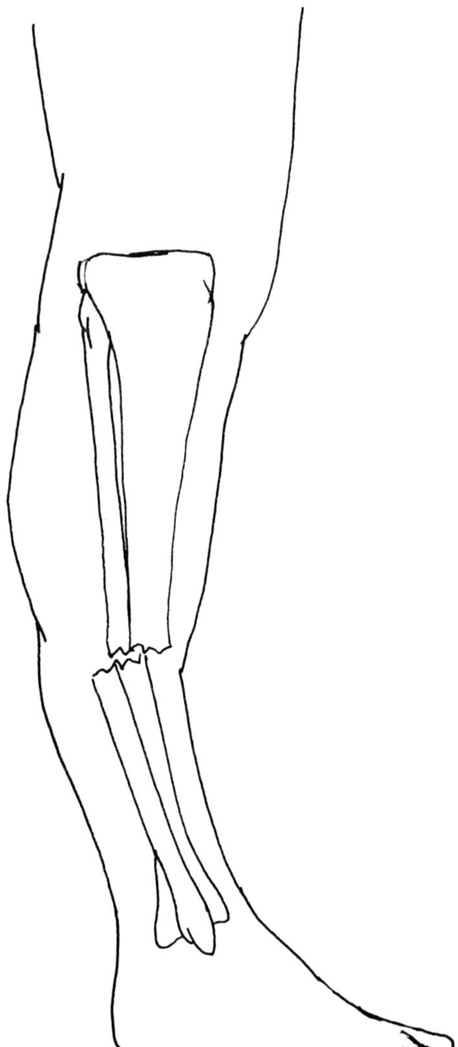

Fig. 1-8. Angulation.

PART I

The Spine

Larry S. Eisenfeld
Sam W. Wiesel

2
The Cervical Spine

Injuries or potential injuries to the cerival spine deserve the respect of every physician examining such a patient. Injuries of the cervical spine can consist of fractures or dislocations causing death, quadriplegia, paraplegia, or having absolutely no neurologic effect. Certainly, lesser injuries such as cervical strain can occur as well. It is imperative that the examining physician carefully scrutinize every cervical spine film not only for fractures but for dislocations and for signs of ligamentous injuries. The routine views consist of lateral view (Fig. 2-1A), anteroposterior (AP) view (Fig. 2-1B), open-mouthed view (Figure 2-1C), and oblique views (Fig. 2-1D). The most important of these views is the lateral view, as it will reveal the majority of unstable injuries and dislocations. Certain key relationships must be checked on every lateral cervical spine film. We have

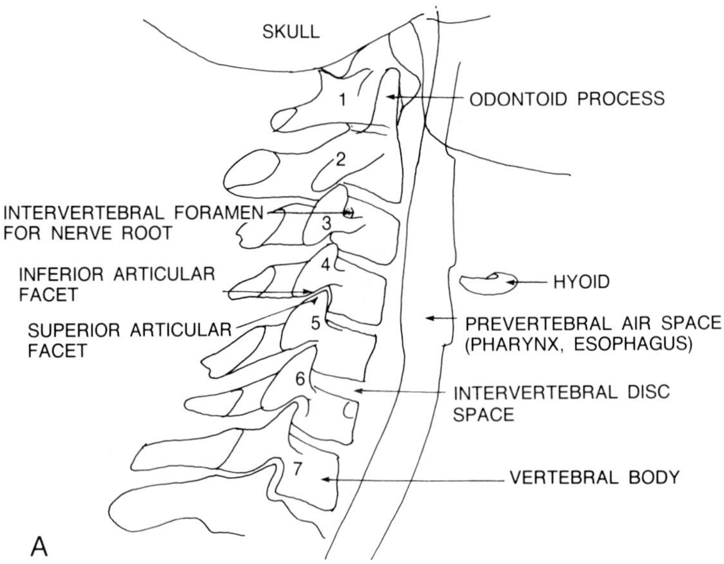

A

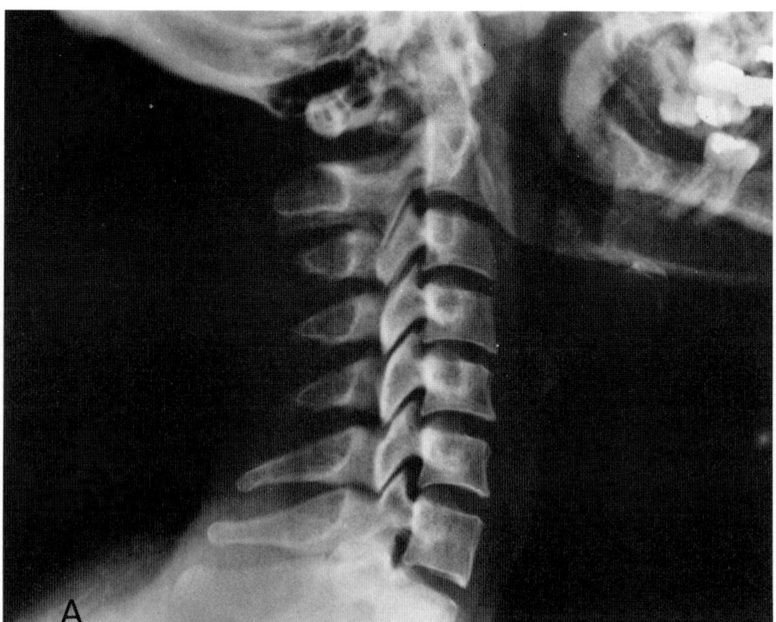

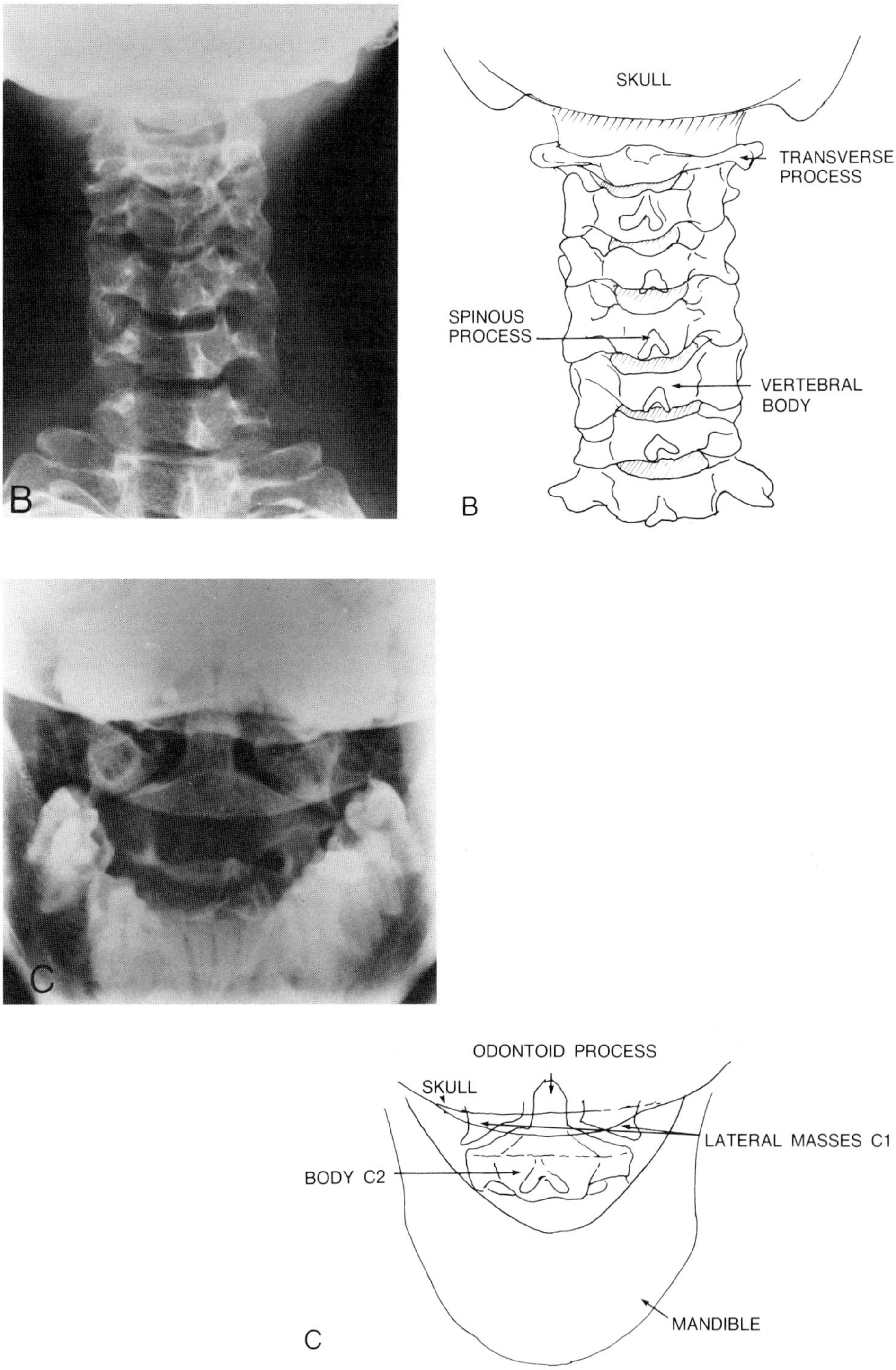

Fig. 2-1. (A) Lateral cervical spine — normal. (B) AP cervical spine — normal. (C) Open-mouthed view, cervical spine — normal (Figure continues).

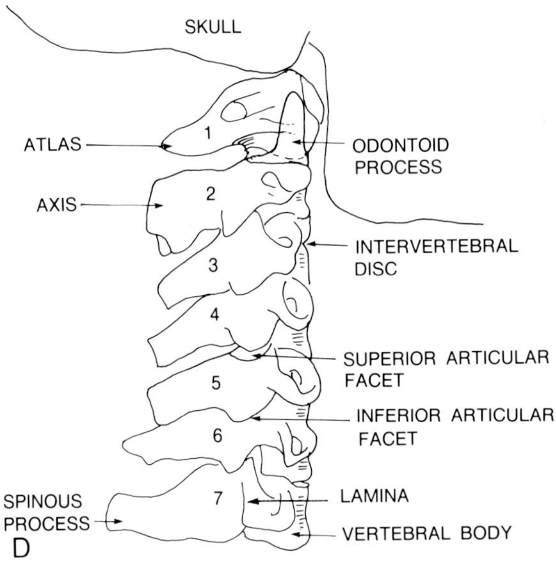

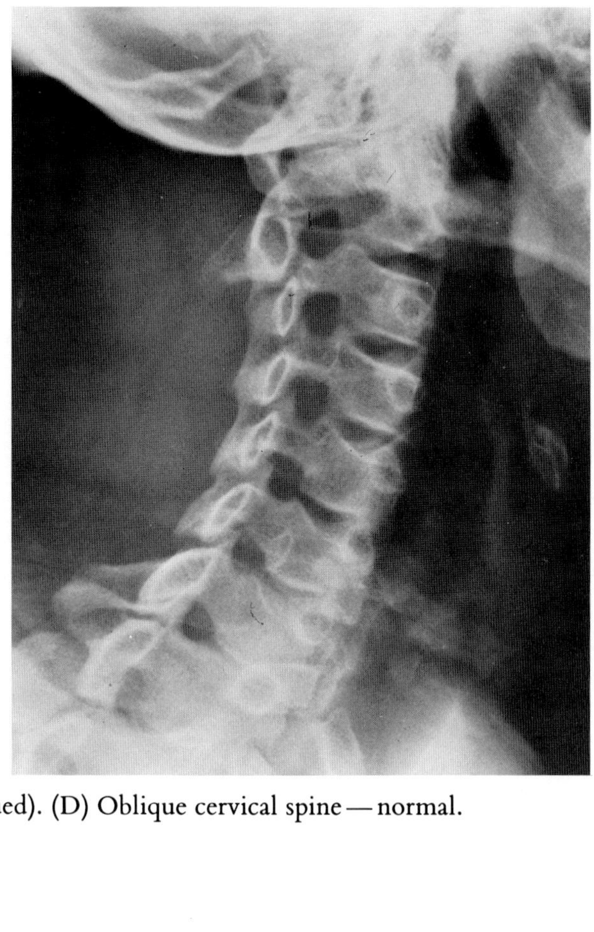

D

Fig. 2-1 (Continued). (D) Oblique cervical spine — normal.

composed the following check list for review of every lateral cervical spine film.

1. A smooth line should be able to be drawn along the anterior/posterior vertebral body border. A 0 to 3.5 mm anterior subluxation may be normal (Fig. 2-2).

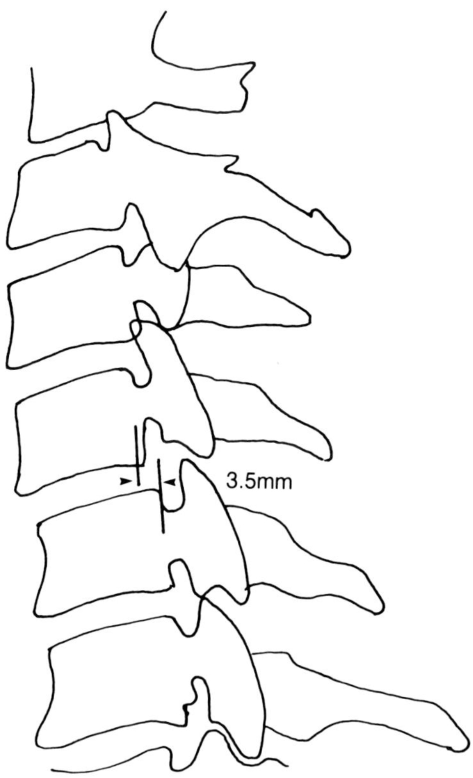

Fig. 2-2. Normal horizontal translation. 3.5 mm of horizontal translation or subluxation of one vertebra upon another may be normal.

2. The odontoid process should be seen below the basion. It should be less than 5 mm in vertical distance and less than 1 mm of horizontal translation from the basion (Fig. 2-3).
3. The retropharangeal space should be no greater than 3 mm away from C3 and no greater than 6 mm away from C5. A greater distance may represent bleeding in the retropharangeal space, secondary to fractures or ligamentous injuries (Fig. 2-3).

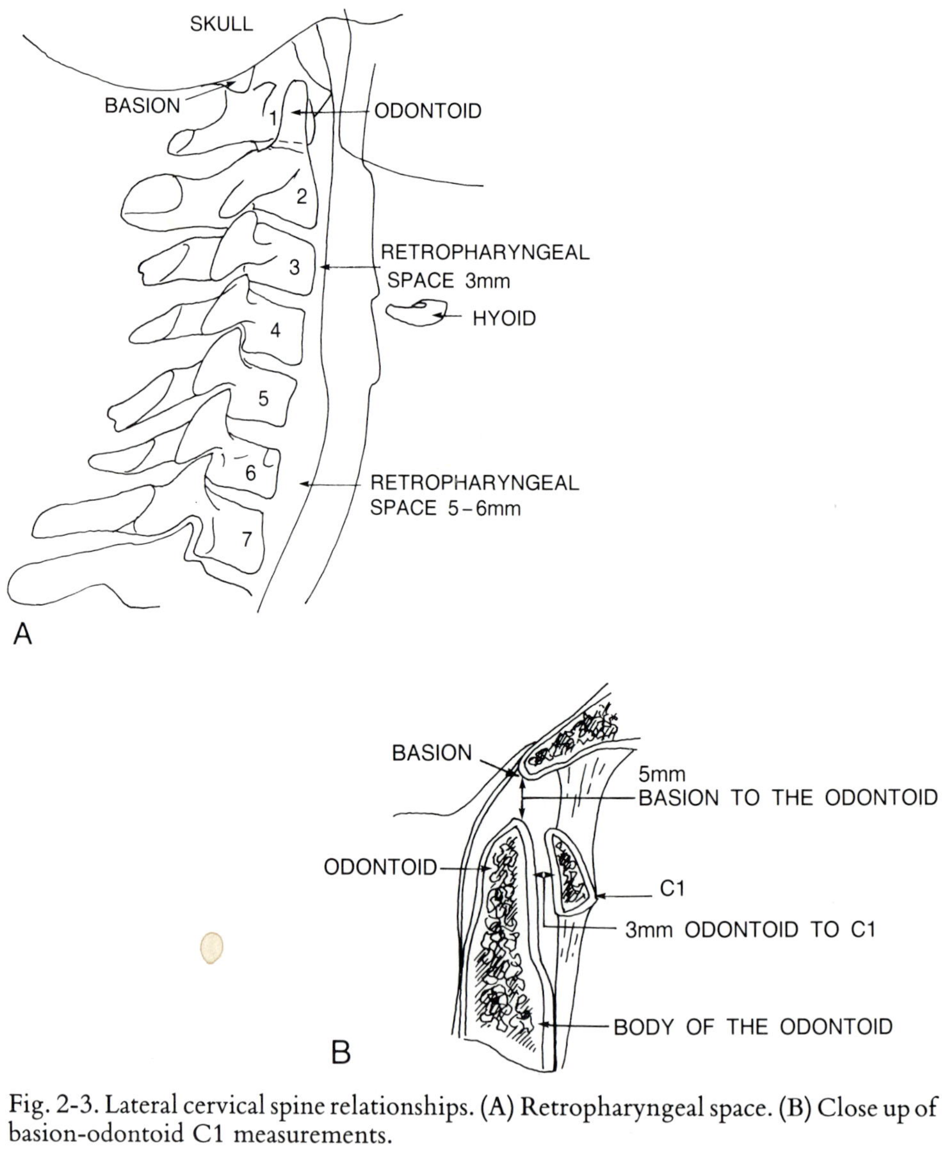

Fig. 2-3. Lateral cervical spine relationships. (A) Retropharyngeal space. (B) Close up of basion-odontoid C1 measurements.

4. An angle of greater than 11° between adjacent vertebral bodies may represent an unstable spine (Fig. 2-4).
5. On the open-mouthed view, it is essential to see that the odontoid is centered between the lateral masses of C1 and that the lateral masses of C1 are aligned over the facet joints of C2 (Fig. 2-1C).

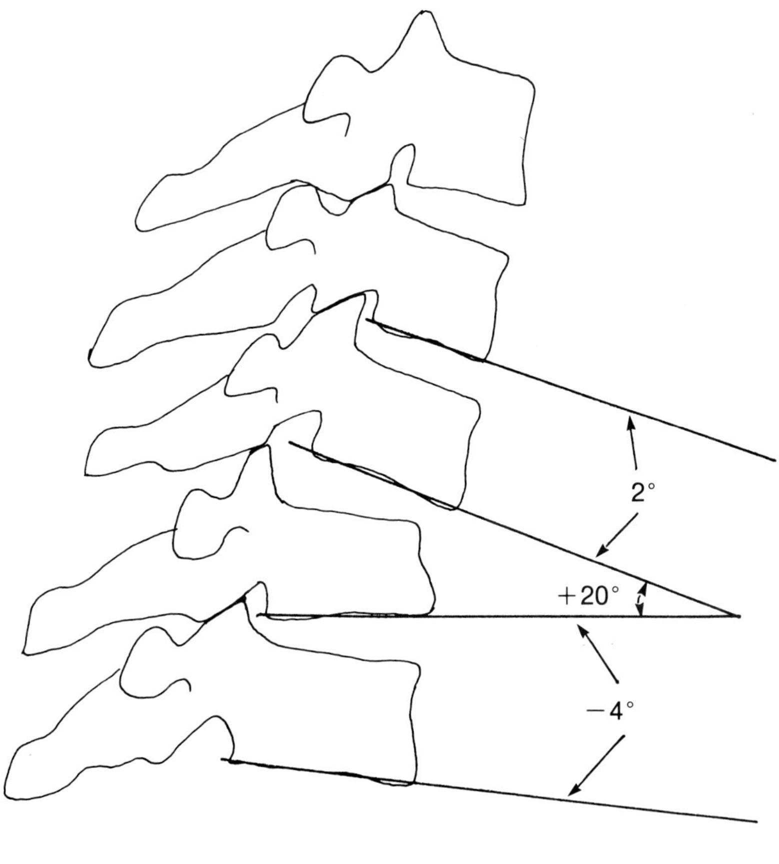

Fig. 2-4. Cervical spine instability. An angle greater than 11 degrees, as measured above, depicts spinal instability.

Jefferson Fracture

This fracture is a break in the osseous ring of C1 and accounts for 2 to 13 percent of cervical spine fractures.

MECHANISM

The fracture is the result of indirect violence, usually resulting from a blow to the vertex or a fall on the head. The weakest part in the arch of C1 is the posterior segment; it usually fractures with the neck in slight extension. Flexion favors fracture of the anterior arch.

CLINICAL PRESENTATION

The patient presents with a stiff neck, inability to nod or rotate the head, and sits as if holding a weight on the head, refusing to move the head. He may localize pain to the occipital and suboccipital areas. In the patient with pain localized to this area, the index of suspicion for the cervical spine injuries should be very high. Neurologic deficit is rare in non-fatal injuries.

ROENTGENOGRAMS

Lateral and open-mouthed views are essential (Fig. 2-5). The lateral roentgenograms may reveal an increase in the retropharyngeal soft tissue space. The open-mouthed view may reveal a spread in the lateral masses, which if greater than 7 mm, is indicative of instability (Fig. 2-6). Flexion and extension roentgenograms should not be done in emergency settings.

COMPLICATIONS

One-third of the patients have associated odontoid or other cervical spine fractures.

TREATMENT

This fracture requires immobilization with a skeletal fixation device such as, "the halo," which is most frequently used.

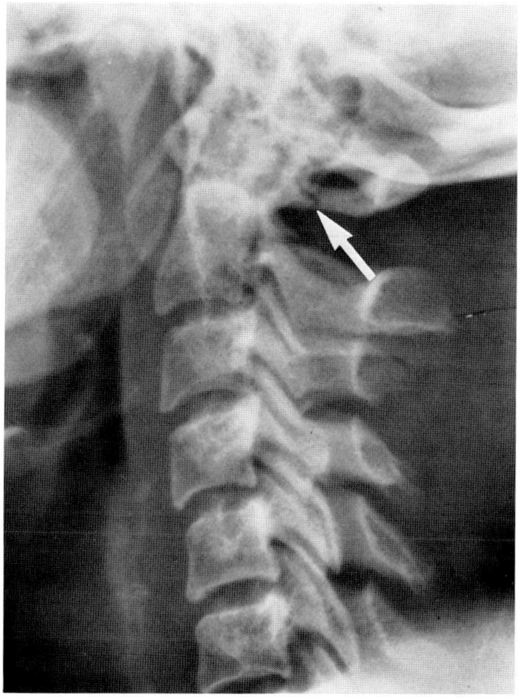

Fig. 2-5. Jefferson fracture (C1). There is a fracture in the posterior arch of C1.

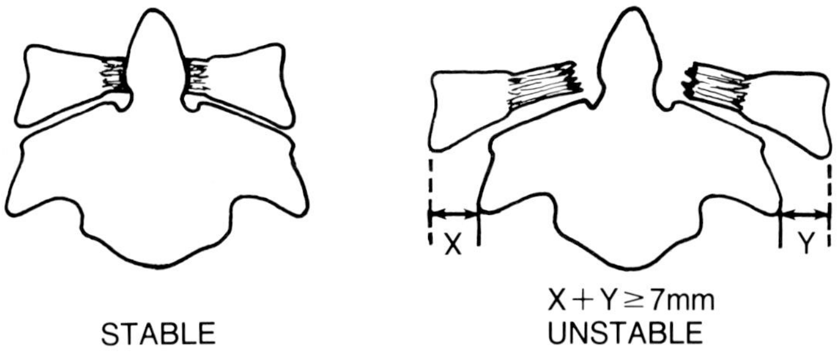

Fig. 2-6. Cervical spine instability in Jefferson fracture is present if X + Y is greater than, or equal to, 7 mm.

Odontoid Fractures

A fracture through the odontoid process which does not involve the axis is called an odontoid fracture. Odontoid fractures have been classified into three types which help in predicting prognosis, healing, and stability (Fig. 2-7). Type 1: There is avulsion of the apex of the odontoid — a very rare injury. Type 2: A fracture at the base of the odontoid without involvement of the body of C2. This is unstable and has the highest rate of non-union. Type 3: A fracture of the body of C2; it is more stable than Type 2.

MECHANISM

A combination of hyperextension and horizontal translation is the etiology of this injury.

CLINICAL PRESENTATION

The patient may relate a feeling of impending doom and may present with hands supporting the chin and occiput as if to prevent the head from "falling off." Pain may be localized to the occipital and suboccipital areas and is often accompanied by neck stiffness and spasm. There is usually no associated neurological deficit.

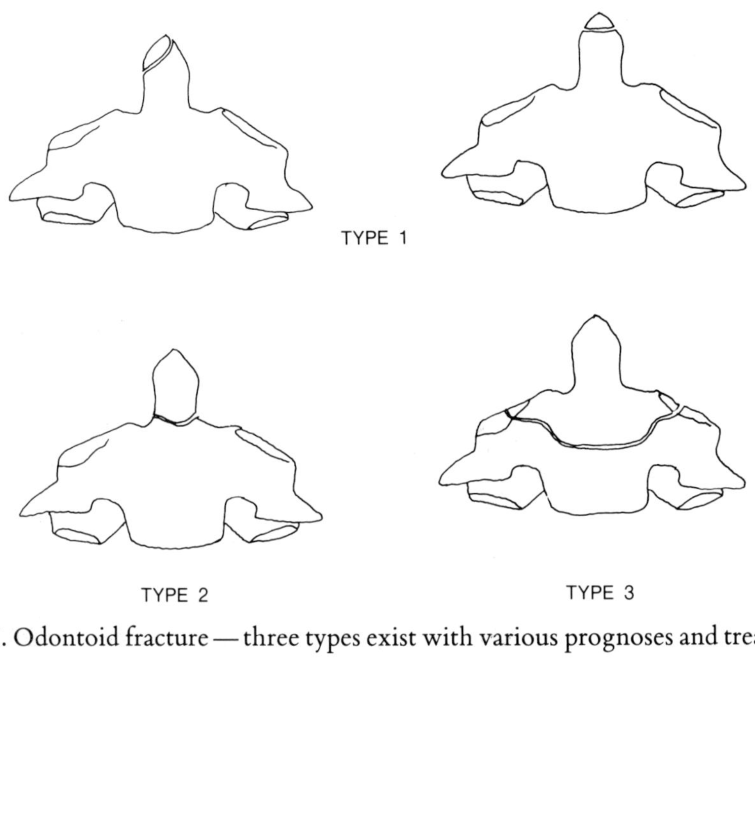

Fig. 2-7. Odontoid fracture — three types exist with various prognoses and treatments.

ROENTGENOGRAMS

The open-mouthed view (Fig. 2-8A) often reveals the fracture. The lateral view (Fig. 2-8B) will confirm whether or not there is any displacement of the fracture. If the index of suspicion is high, and the routine films are negative, tomograms are indicated.

TREATMENT

Type 1 fractures may be treated with a Philadelphia hard collar. For Type 2 and Type 3 fractures, skeletal immobilization is recommended as quickly as possible.

A
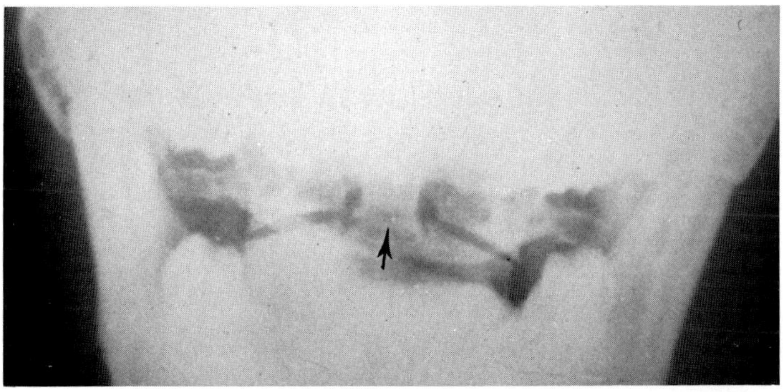

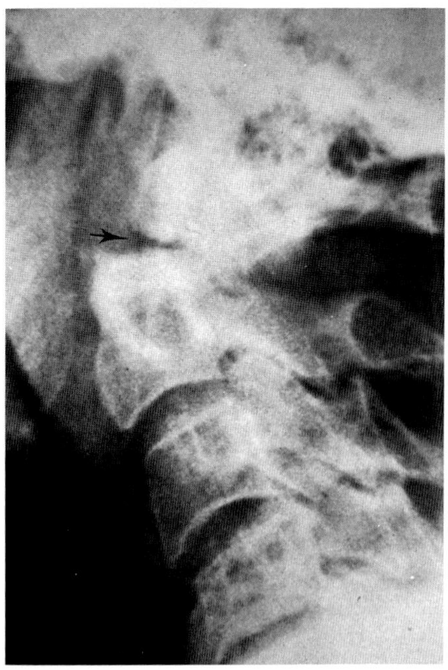
B

Fig. 2-8. Odontoid fracture. (A) Open mouth view. (B) Lateral view. This is a nondisplaced fracture.

Hangman's Fracture

This eponym is used to describe a bilateral neural arch fracture of the axis (C2) without an odontoid fracture.

MECHANISM

Although the description correctly suggests the fracture may arise from a hanging, it is now commonly due to high speed automobile accidents in which a combination of hyperextension and axial compression are responsible for the injury.

CLINICAL PRESENTATION

The patient complains of neck stiffness and refuses to move the neck. He gives a history of a compressive blow to the vertex. Neurological injury is uncommon because of the wide diameter of the spinal canal at this level.

ROENTGENOGRAMS

AP and lateral roentgenograms (Fig. 2-9) will reveal the neural arch fracture and whether or not subluxation is present. Subluxation is indicative of injury to the anterior or posterior longitudinal ligaments.

COMPLICATIONS

The fracture is unstable but heals readily with adequate immobilization. Associated fracture may be present in the lower cervical spine.

TREATMENT

Skeletal immobilization.

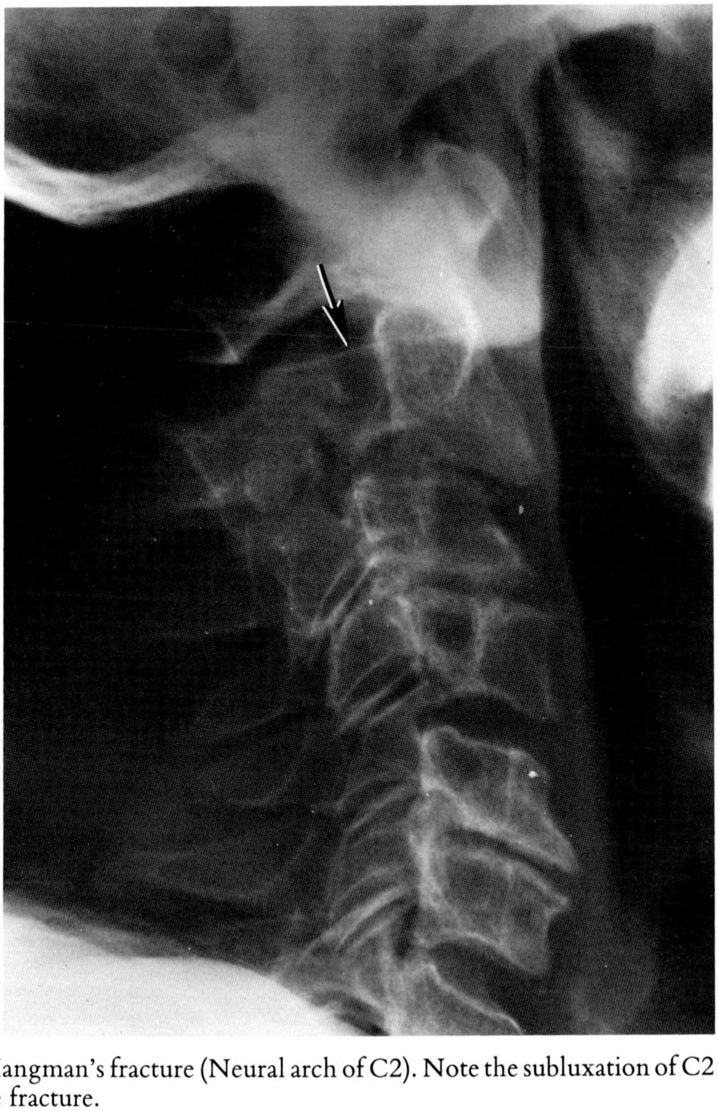

Fig. 2-9. Hangman's fracture (Neural arch of C2). Note the subluxation of C2 on C3, as well as the fracture.

"Burst" Fracture

MECHANISM

Direct axial compression with the head in slight extension produces a "bursting" of the vertebral body. The most common level of injury is C5.

CLINICAL PRESENTATION

The patient often presents with a neurological deficit as a result of posterior protrusion of bone or of disc material into the spinal canal. A high incidence of neurological complications requires that this patient be carefully evaluated by an orthopaedic surgeon or neurosurgeon for full evaluation of the injury and skeletal immobilization.

ROENTGENOGRAMS

AP, lateral, and oblique roentgenograms will demonstrate the fracture. An avulsion of the anterior inferior surface has been characteristically called a "tear-drop" fracture (Fig. 2-10). This is actually a type of "burst" fracture. The serious problem associated with these fractures is caused by bone and/or disc material protruded into the spinal canal, causing cord compression. Although these injuries may appear relatively harmless, they may have very serious sequelae, including quadriplegia.

COMPLICATIONS

Neurological injury is quite variable, depending upon the position and the amount of protruded material. Concomitant cervical spine fractures as well as closed head injuries may also be present.

TREATMENT

In the presence of neurological deficit, immediate evaluation by an orthopaedist or a neurosurgeon is recommended. Skeletal immobilization is mandatory.

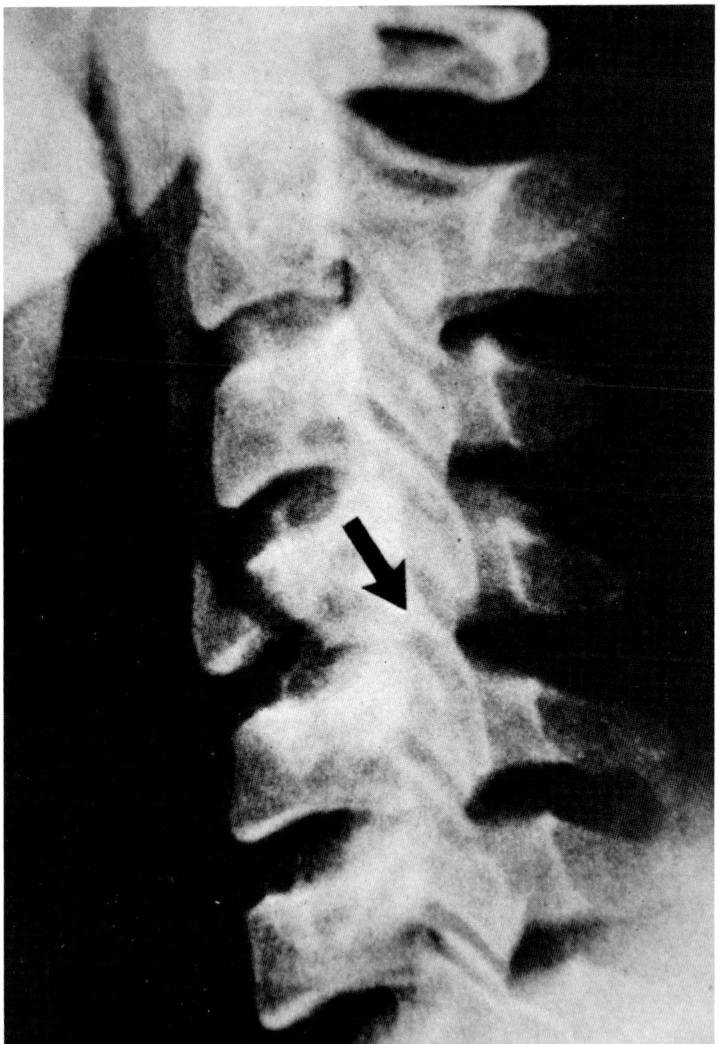

Fig. 2-10. Teardrop (Burst) fracture. There is displacement of the anterior-inferior portion of the vertebral body. The arrow indicates the relationships of the facet joint.

"Clay-Shoveler's" Fracture

This fracture is an avulsion of one or more of the lower cervical or upper thoracic spinous processes.

MECHANISM

The fracture is due to forceful contracture of the muscles attaching to the posterior spinous process, most commonly at C7.

CLINICAL PRESENTATION

The patient presents with pain, stiffness in the neck, and tenderness which may be localized to the level of the avulsion fracture.

ROENTGENOGRAMS

Lateral cervical roentgenograms (Fig. 2-11), best show the avulsion of the spinous process. It is a safe, stable fracture.

TREATMENT

Symptomatic, with analgesics and a soft collar.

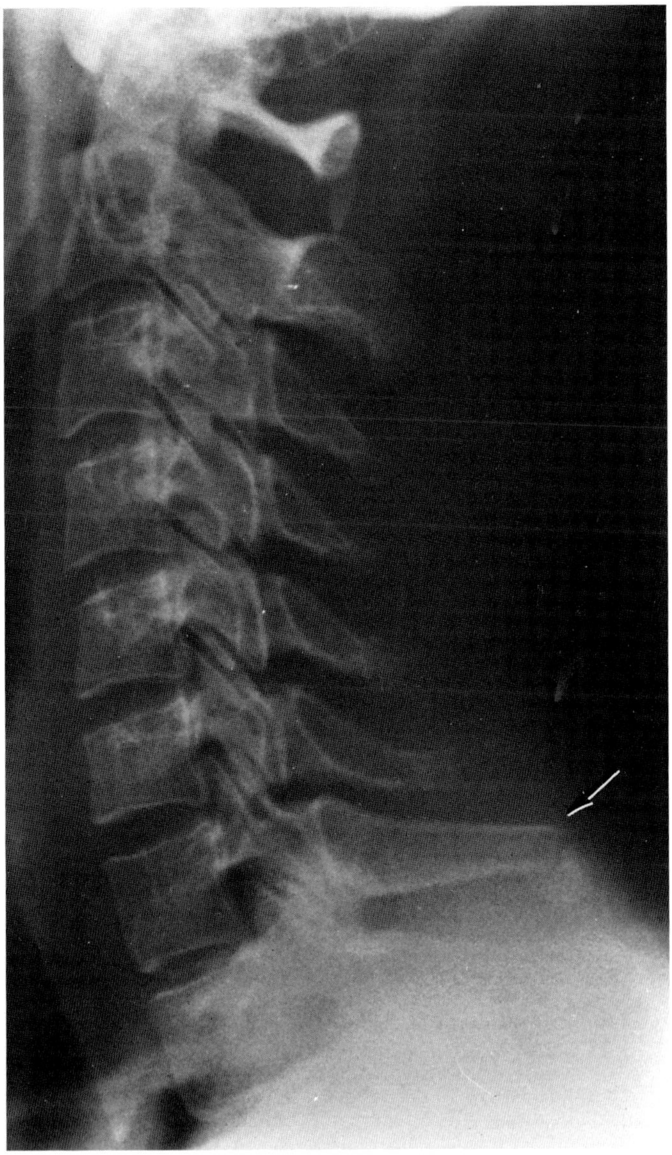

Fig. 2-11. Clayshoveler's fracture. An avulsion fracture of the spinous process of C7 (arrow).

Occipital-Atlanto (C1) Instability

A complete occipital-atlanto dislocation is usually a fatal injury.

MECHANISM

A violent, twisting force to the head is usually the mechanism of injury. The degree of ligamentous injury determines the degree of instability of this joint.

CLINICAL PRESENTATION

The patient may present with pain and swelling in the neck and there may be no neurological deficit.

ROENTGENOGRAMS

Lateral roentgenograms are necessary for evaluating this injury. The lateral roentgenogram (Fig. 2-12) may reveal an increase in the retropharyngeal soft tissue space. The basion-odontoid relationship must be evaluated. Clinical instability is suggested if there is a horizontal translation of the odontoid below the basion greater than 1 mm or if there is a vertical distance between the odontoid and basion of greater than 5 mm (Fig. 2-3). Flexion-extension views should not be obtained in the emergency room.

COMPLICATIONS

Due to the highly unstable nature of this injury, treatment with skeletal traction may actually increase the displacement. Concomitant cervical spine trauma may also be present as well as closed head injuries.

TREATMENT

Skeletal immobilization and careful application of traction. Roentgenograms must be taken once traction is applied.

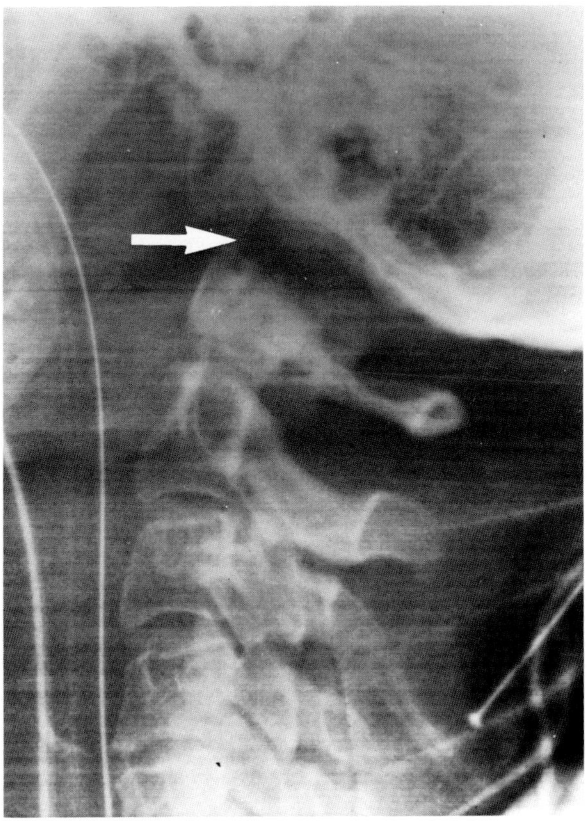

Fig. 2-12. Occipital-atlanto instability. Note the increased space between the odointoid and the basion.

Atlanto-Axial Instability (C1-C2)

This is an injury to the transverse ligament leading to instability of the C1-C2 articulations.

MECHANISM

Four different mechanisms, each causing a different injury, have been identified. 1. Anterior dislocation—This injury is usually fatal because the cord is severely injured by compression between the neural arch posteriorly and an intact odontoid process. 2. Anterior dislocation plus an odontoid fracture—neurologic damage is variable, depending upon the extent of the injury. 3. Posterior dislocation—this is a rare lesion due to a sudden extension of the head or a blow to the submental area. The atlas is dislocated posterior to the odontoid. 4. Rotatory subluxation—this facet injury may produce irreducible torticollis if unilateral (possibly death if bilateral). The severity of lesions can be related to the extent of the ligamentous injury.

CLINICAL PRESENTATION

As mentioned above, clinical presentation is variable. Pain and swelling of the neck are present with any type of movement.

ROENTGENOGRAMS

The lateral roentgenogram is the most important (Fig. 2-13). On it, careful measurements need to be made to ascertain the relationship of the posterior arch of C1 to the anterior surface of the odontoid. The normal distance between C1 and C2 is 0 to 3 mm. This implies that the transverse ligaments are intact. A subluxation of 3 to 5 mm is indicative of rupture of the transverse ligament. Subluxation greater than 5 mm correlates with rupture of both the transverse and alar ligaments. This situation depicts an unstable spine.

COMPLICATIONS

Fractures of the lower cervical spine and closed head injuries may also be present.

TREATMENT

Reduction of the subluxation and skeletal immobilization are needed as emergency treatment.

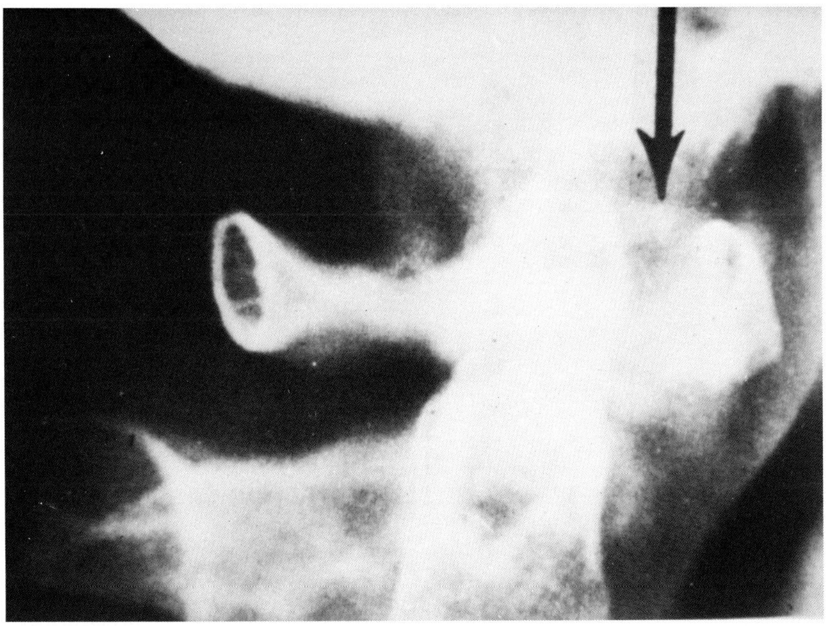

Fig. 2-13. Atlanto-axial (C1-C2 instability). Note the marked space between C1 and C2.

Lower Cervical Spine Subluxation and Dislocation

The combination of hyperflexion and rotation is a common mechanism for dislocation or subluxation in the lower cervical spine.

CLINICAL PRESENTATION

The neck may be stiff and painful. Unilateral facet dislocation may be accompanied by symptoms of nerve root compression. There is usually no sign of cord injury, although in rare cases the Brown-Sequard syndrome may be present. Bilateral facet dislocation may present with symptoms of cord compression and frequently is accompanied by quadriplegia.

ROENTGENOGRAMS

AP and lateral roentgenograms (Fig. 2-14) are essential to evaluate the degree of subluxation. Oblique roentgenograms are often helpful to better detect a facet fracture and loss of the normal facet articulations. Occasionally, tomograms are necessary. The essential evaluation is to be made on the lateral roentgenograms (Fig. 2-15). A subluxation of 25 percent of one vertebral body on the other is seen with a unilateral facet dislocation. A subluxation of 50 percent or greater is seen with bilateral facet dislocation and is an unstable injury. In association with facet dislocation, one may see an angular deformity of the vertebral bodies. This may be due to either a facet fracture or ligamentous injury. Lateral flexion extension roentgenograms may be necessary to elucidate this condition, but need not be done in the emergency room.

COMPLICATIONS

Neurologic deficit may range from no injury to quadriplegia. In bilateral facet dislocation, stability is inversely proportional to the ease of reduction (i.e., the easier the reduction, the less stable the fracture and the greater the need for fixation).

TREATMENT

Reduction of the dislocation is essential. The unilateral facet dislocation is usually stable once reduced. Often, bilateral facet dislocations are unstable and require additional fixation.

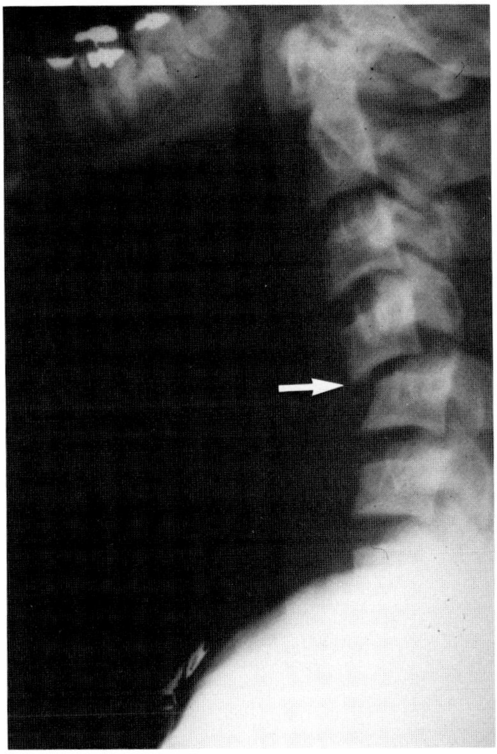

Fig. 2-14. Cervical spine subluxation —C4 on C5.

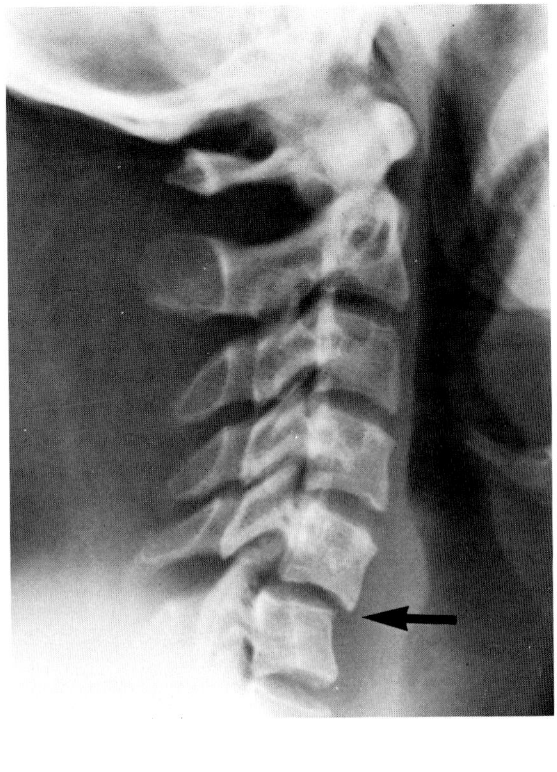

Fig. 2-15. Unilateral facet dislocation. Here the horizontal translation equals 1/4 of the depth of the vertebral body. The arrow indicates the facet dislocation.

Cervical Strain

Neck pain, stiffness, and the absence of positive findings on roentgenograms are usually due to paravertebral muscle spasm. If there is associated arm pain, the possibility of cervical disc protrusion or nerve root avulsion must be entertained. These are non-emergency problems and need symptomatic relief of pain, cervical collar, bedrest, mild analgesics, and the appropriate follow-up.

"Whiplash" is a hyperextension injury usually caused by "rear-end" motor vehicle accidents. This injury has been greatly reduced with the advent of high seat backs and head rests which block hyperextension of the neck. The injury is to the soft tissues of the neck and the appropriate treatment is symptomatic. Roentgenograms in both of these situations are usually normal, although one may see straightening of the normal lordosis, which is a non-specific finding.

3
The Thoracolumbar Spine

The ribs attach to the thoracic vertebrae to form a protective shell around the vital, intrathoracic organs. The routine AP view (Fig. 3-1A) and lateral view (Fig. 3-1B) will reveal most fractures or dislocations in the thoracic spine. "Coned-down" views of the area in question may give greater clarity of the vertebrae involved. With the stability added by the ribs, thoracic spine dislocations above T10 are uncommon.

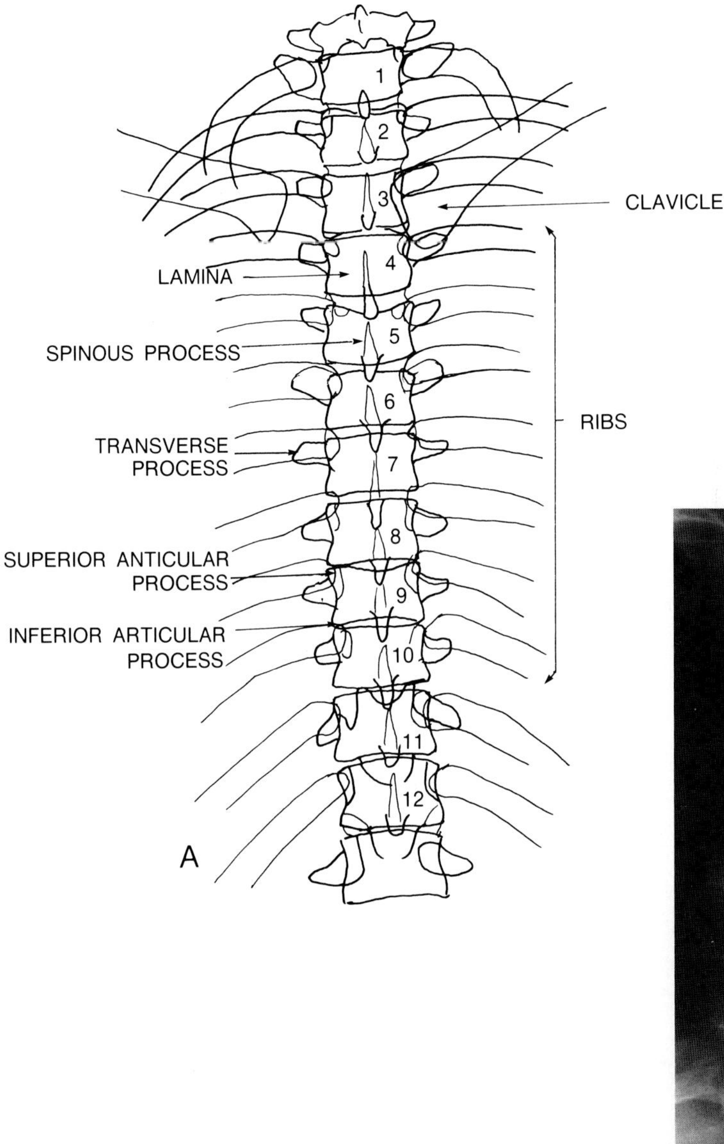

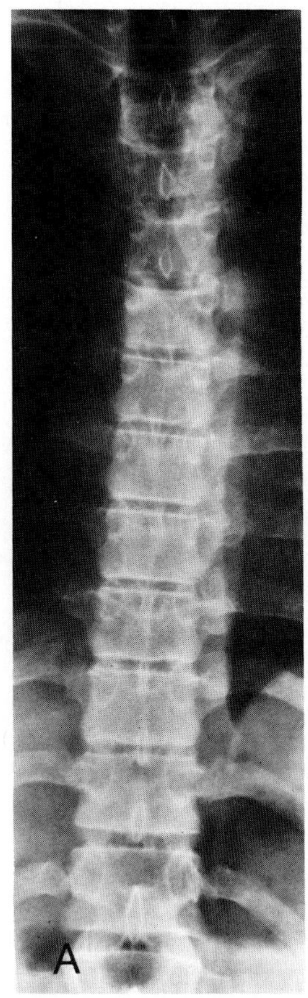

Fig. 3-1. (A) (Figure continues).

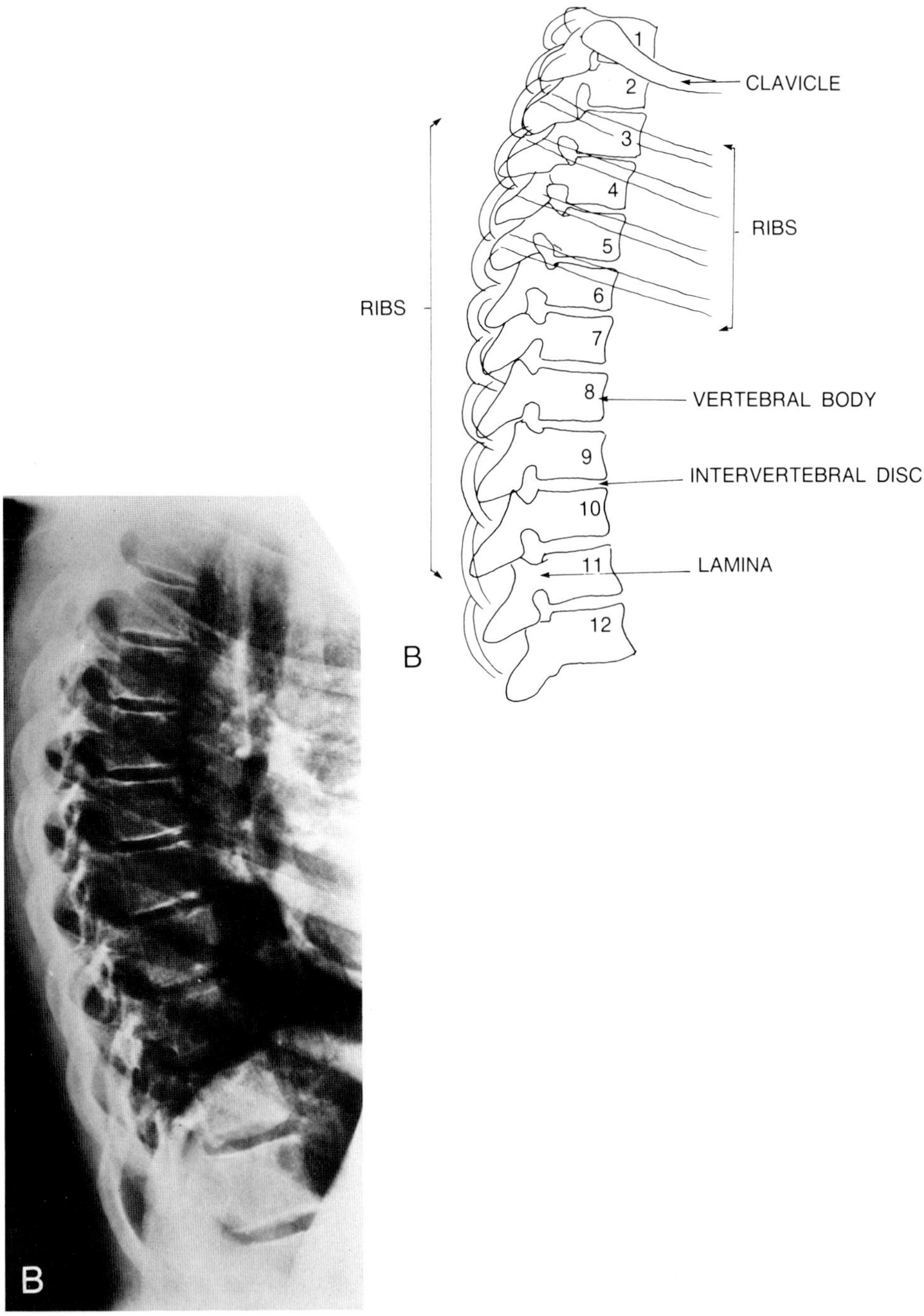

Fig. 3-1. (A) AP thoracic spine — normal. (B) Lateral thoracic spine — normal.

The lumbar spine requires an AP view (Fig. 3-2A), lateral view (Fig. 3-2B), oblique views (Fig. 3-2C), and a "spot" lateral of L4-S1 (Fig. 3-2D) for a complete study. Due to the change in vertebral configuration between the thoracic and lumbar vertebra, most thoracolumbar dislocations occur between T10 and L2. Neurologic damage occurs with 60 to 70 percent of fractures or fracture dislocations of the thoracolumbar spine. In patients with a pure dislocation, neurologic damage approaches 100 percent. The treating physician needs to be alert for the highly unstable spine which may spontaneously reduce to anatomic position when the patient is supine for radiographic studies. Obviously, concern for intrathoracic and intra-abdominal structures should be very high.

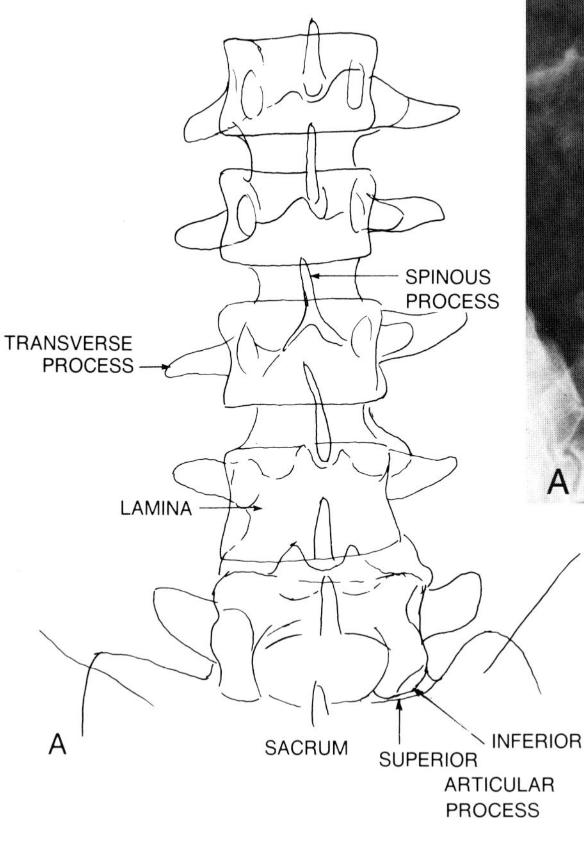

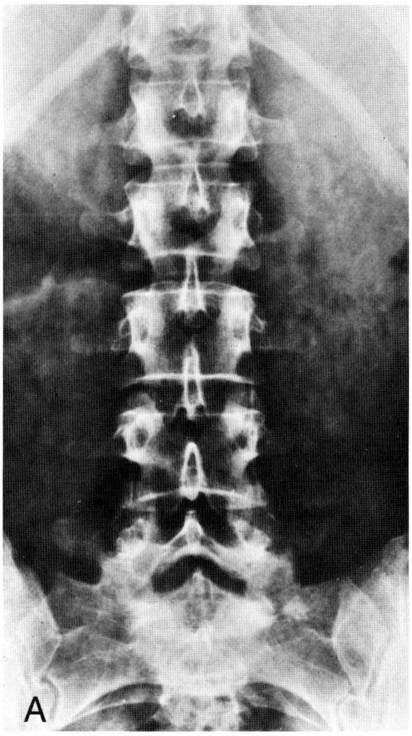

Fig. 3-2. (A) (Figure continues).

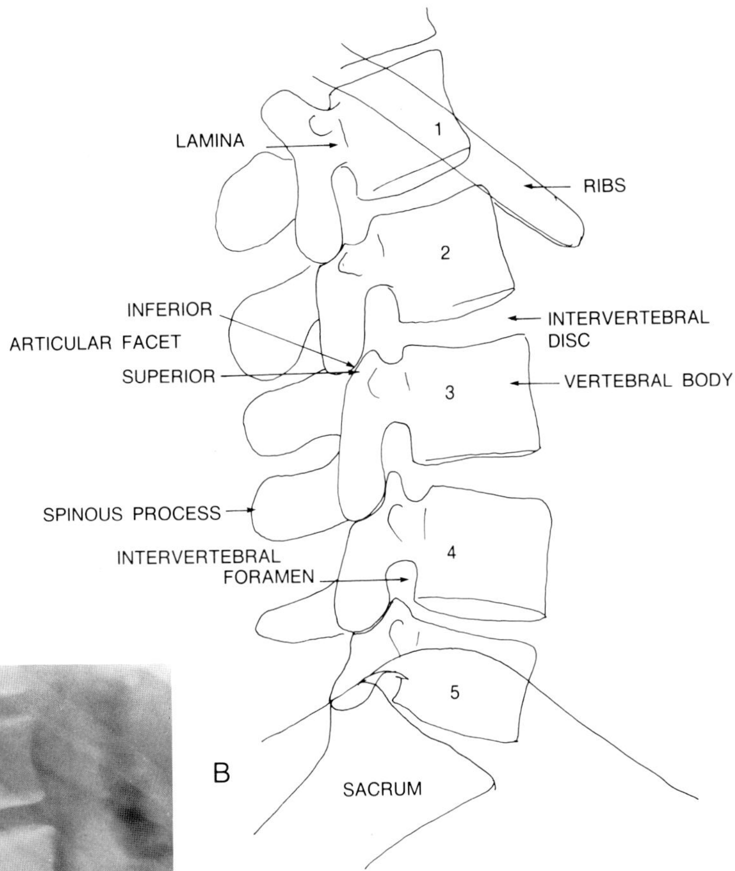

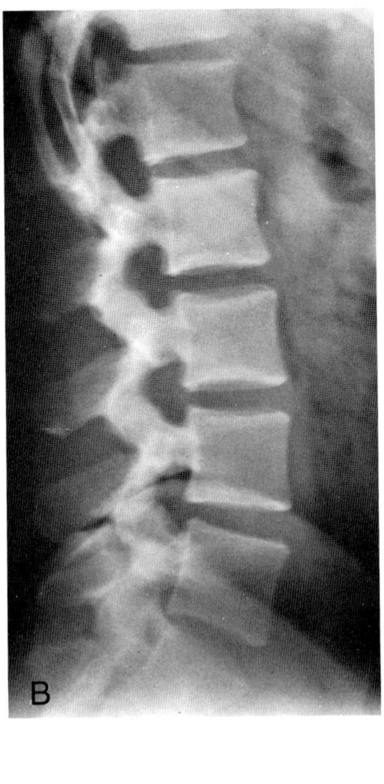

Fig. 3-2. (B) (Figure continues).

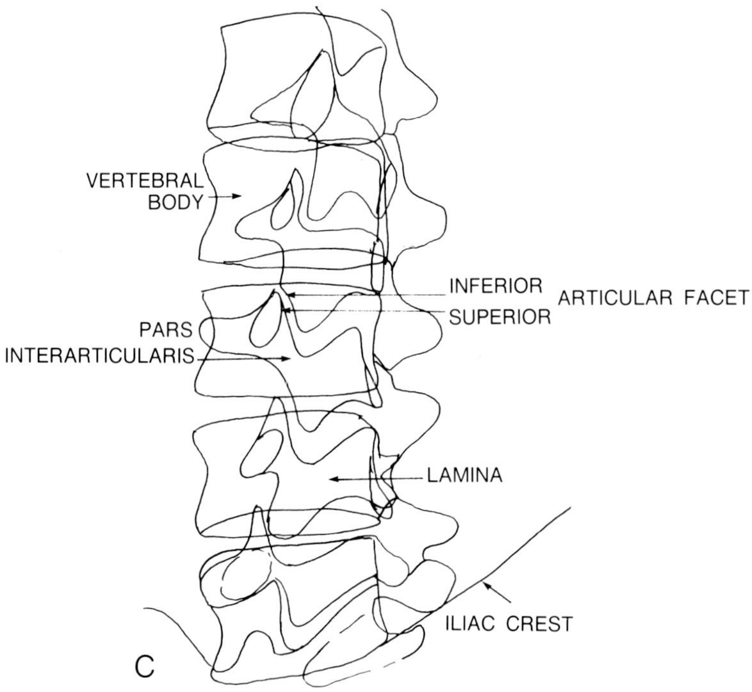

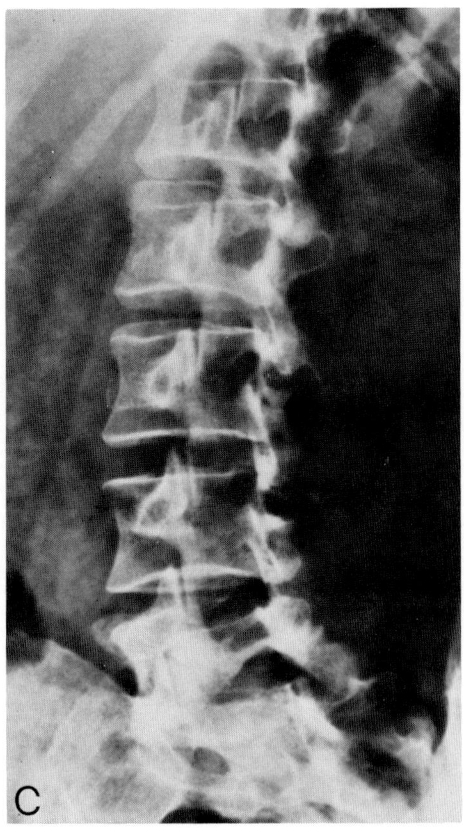

Fig. 3-2. (A) AP lumbar spine — normal. (B) Lateral lumbar spine — normal. (C) Oblique lumbar spine — normal. (D) "Spot view" of L5-S1 — normal.

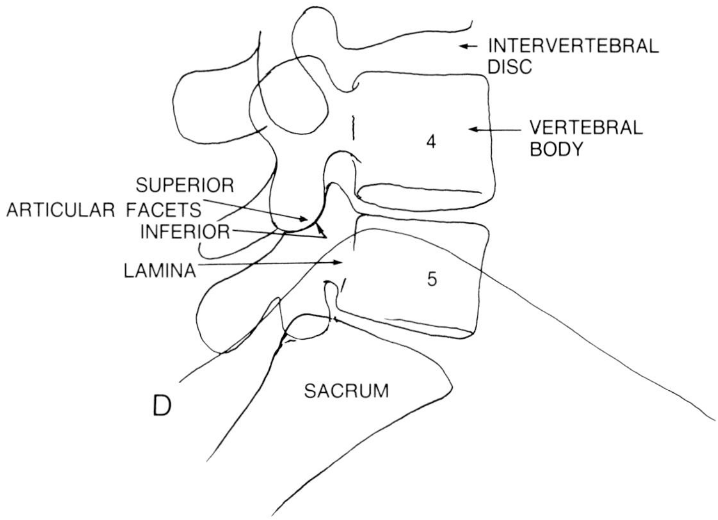
INTERVERTEBRAL
DISC
VERTEBRAL
BODY
4
5
SUPERIOR
ARTICULAR FACETS
INFERIOR
LAMINA
SACRUM

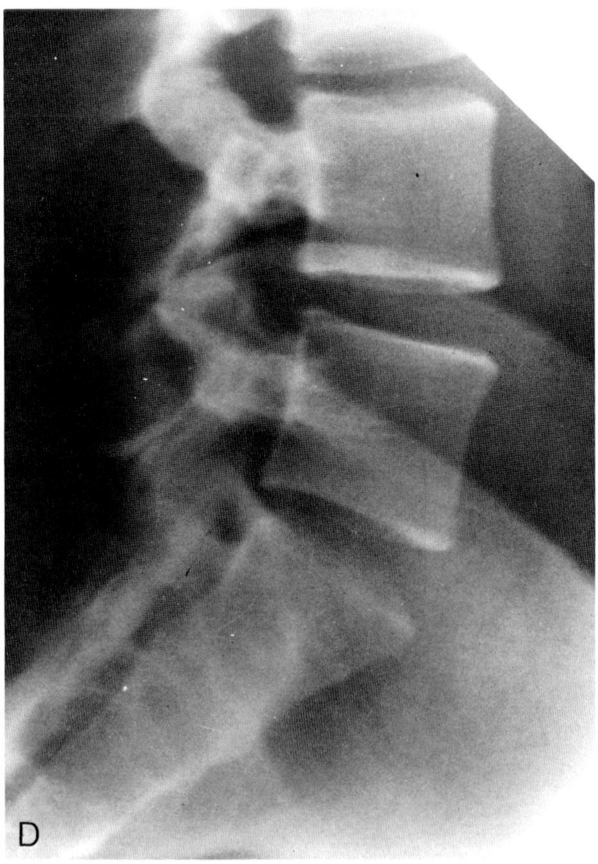

Fig. 3-2. (D)

Thoracolumbar Fracture Dislocation

Sixty to 65 percent of these injuries result in paraplegia due to cord and cauda-equina injuries. The neurologic deficit due to cauda-equina injury may decrease with time and return to normal.

MECHANISM

This injury is always a combination of rotation with another force, either flexion or extension. The rotatory forces tear the ligaments that are crucial for spine stability, and it is the flexion and extension forces that cause the fracture.

CLINICAL PRESENTATION

Sixty to 65 percent of these patients present with neurological loss due to cord or cauda-equina injuries. Back pain is uniformly present.

ROENTGENOGRAMS

AP and lateral roentgenograms (Fig. 3-3) are usually satisfactory for evaluating this injury. It is again emphasized that a highly unstable fracture may spontaneously reduce when the patient is supine. The most unstable injury is a horizontal vertebral body fracture, fracture of the articular process, and rupture of all ligaments.

COMPLICATIONS

In approximately two-thirds of patients, associated fractures may be seen in the spine or the lower extremity, depending on the exact mechanism of injury.

TREATMENT

Reduction and immobilization are necessary. Surgery may be necessary, and an Orthopaedic Surgeon or Neurosurgeon should be asked to evaluate the patient.

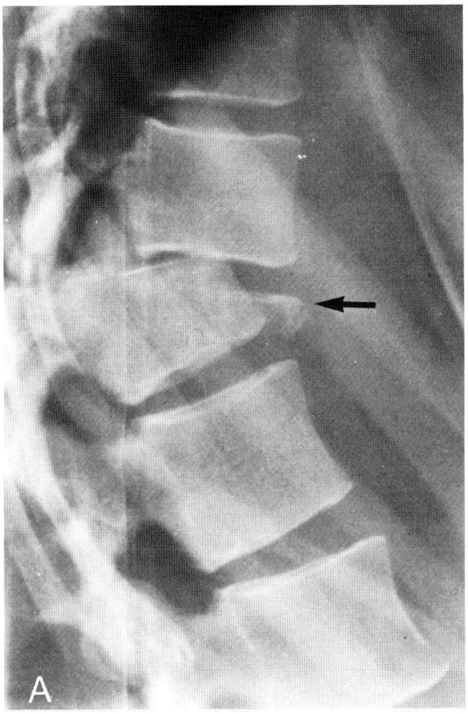

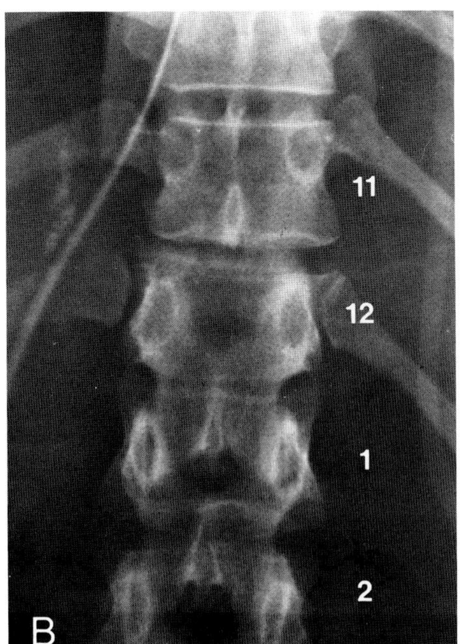

Fig. 3-3. Thoracolumbar fracture dislocation. (A) Lateral T11-12 dislocation. (B) AP view. Note the relatively normal-appearing AP view. The absence of the spinous process of T12 is the only indication that something is abnormal.

Compression Fracture

This is the most frequent thoracolumbar fracture. If trauma is insignificant, it may be the initial sign of an underlying medical problem. The vertebral body may be affected by infection, neoplasia, or metabolic disease, rendering it quite weak. A compression fracture may also be associated with other significant traumatic injuries. However, in any compression fracture caused by minor trauma, the possibility of an underlying process should be investigated.

In clinical practice, the terms "wedge" and "compression" fracture are often used interchangeably. In the pure sense, the mechanism of injury differs, so they are discussed separately in this text.

MECHANISM

These injuries result from a compression force applied to the vertebral body. The intervertebral disc is a more incompressible structure than the vertebral body, and the resultant injury is a fracture of the superior plate of the vertebral body. They are more frequent in elderly patients with severely demineralized bone.

ROENTGENOGRAMS

AP and lateral roentgenograms (Fig. 3-4) should be obtained. A careful search foı other abnormalities of bone should be made if there was only minor trauma. This is felt to be a stable fracture if the anterior compression is less than 50 percent of the vertebral body height.

COMPLICATIONS

Neurological injury is rare. When this fracture is due to a significant trauma such as a fall or a jump, there are frequently other lower extremity injuries such as calcaneal and ankle fractures. It is essential to obtain roentgenograms of the foot and ankle if any complaints of pain are related to this area.

TREATMENT

Investigation for an underlying disease process may be necessary. Initial treatment is bedrest and symptomatic.

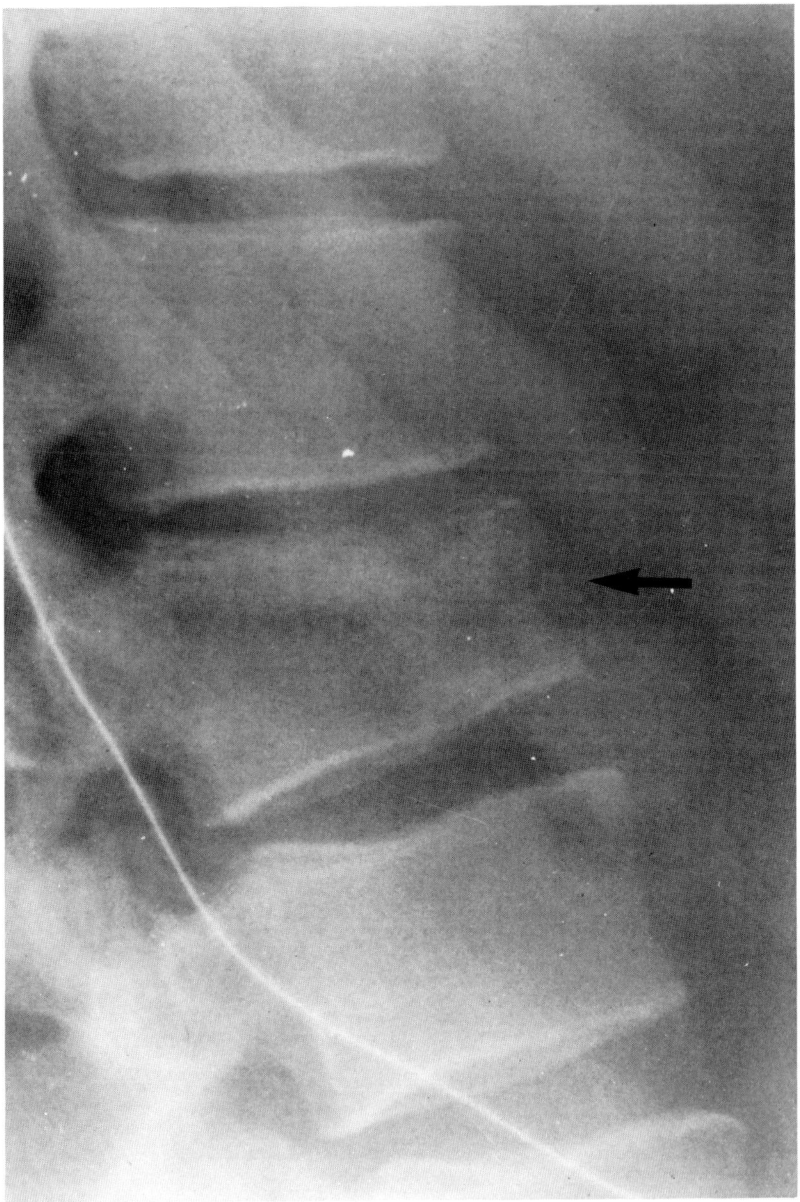

Fig. 3-4. Compression fracture. Check the relationship of the anterior vertebral body height to the posterior vertebral body height. Greater than 50 percent compression of the anterior portion indicates spinal instability.

Wedge Fracture

This fracture is a compression of the anterior portion of the vertebral body with the posterior boundary remaining intact.

MECHANISM

An anterior wedge fracture results from a flexion force. If there is asymmetry of the load in force, a lateral wedge may be produced. Anterior wedge fractures account for 15 percent of spine fractures.

CLINICAL PRESENTATION

Pain in the area of the fracture.

ROENTGENOGRAMS

AP and lateral roentgenograms (Fig. 3-5) are necessary to evaluate this injury. The lateral wedge fracture is often associated with fracture of the transverse process.

COMPLICATIONS

Fracture of the transverse process or other spine fractures may be present. Neurologic damage is more common with the lateral wedge fracture. A significant ileus may follow a wedge fracture.

TREATMENT

Because of the possible associated injuries, these patients should usually be hospitalized with bedrest for symptomatic relief. Ultimately, placement in a brace may be indicated.

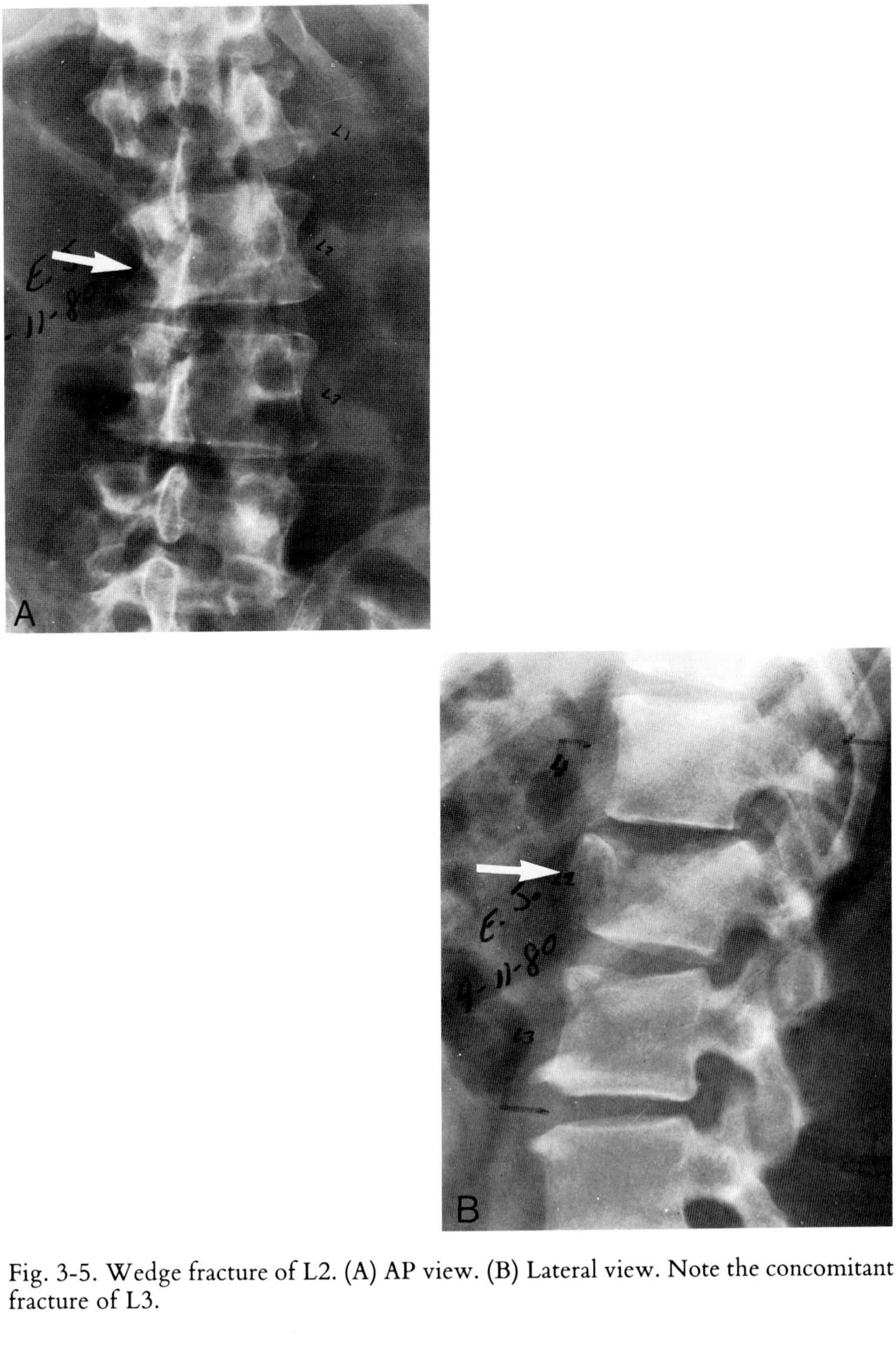

Fig. 3-5. Wedge fracture of L2. (A) AP view. (B) Lateral view. Note the concomitant fracture of L3.

Transverse Process Fracture

MECHANISM

This fracture may be due to a direct blow or an avulsion fracture from the shearing forces by the pull of the psoas muscle or it may be associated with a lateral wedge fracture.

CLINICAL PRESENTATION

This injury requires significant force and may be associated with intra-abdominal injuries. These fractures are locally very painful and tender. The patient resists any motion since this will exacerbate the pain.

ROENTGENOGRAMS

An AP roentgenogram of the spine will reveal the fracture (Fig. 3-6). Other painful and tender areas of the pelvis or lower extremities should also have a radiologic evaluation.

COMPLICATIONS

Due to the significant force required for these injuries, intra-abdominal injuries may occur. There may be significant ileus without intra-abdominal injuries. Renal injuries are also quite common with the transverse process fracture.

TREATMENT

After other injuries have been evaluated, treatment is bedrest and analgesics.

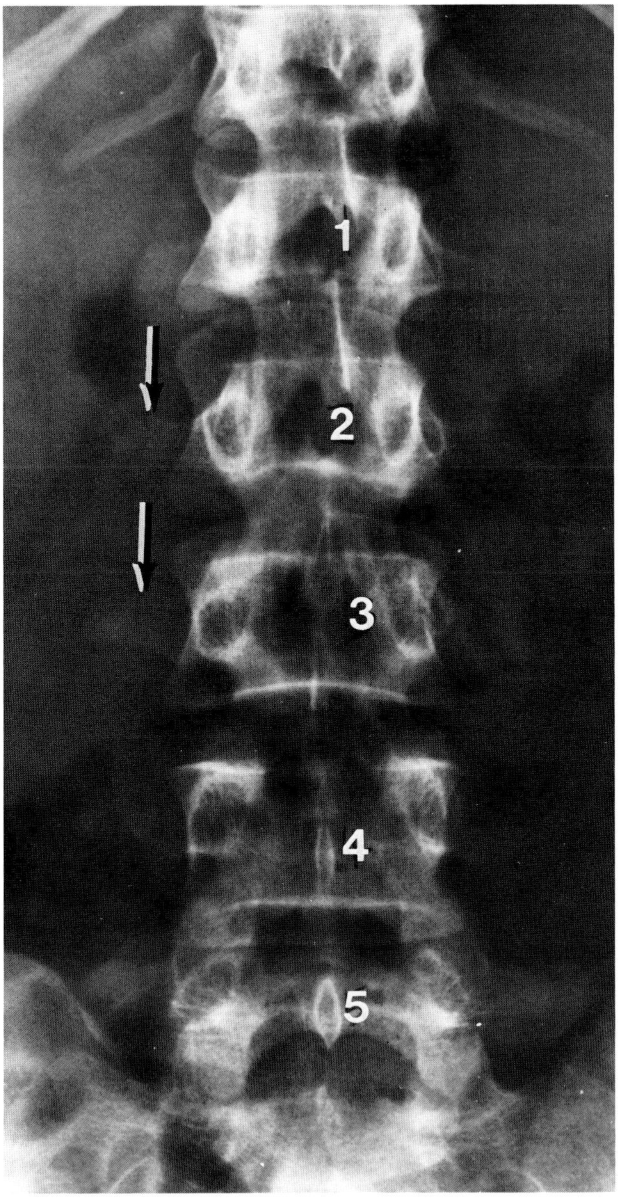

Fig. 3-6. Transverse process fracture — L2 and L3 (arrows).

Chance Fracture

This is a horizontal fracture through the spinous process and vertebral body with posterior ligamentous rupture, subluxation, or fracture of the facet joint.

MECHANISM

This injury results from a combination of flexion and distraction.

CLINICAL PRESENTATION

The patient presents with a variable neurologic deficit in 10 to 15 percent of cases. Back pain and tenderness are uniformly found.

ROENTGENOGRAMS

AP roentgenogram (Fig. 3-7A) reveals a fracture through the pedicles and a tear-shaped appearance of the spinous process. Lateral roentgenograms (Fig. 3-7B) reveal the fracture in the spinous process, and vertebral body. Oblique views add little additional information

COMPLICATIONS

Neurologic injury occurs in 10 to 15 percent of patients, and ileus is frequently associated with these injuries.

TREATMENT

This injury is essentially stable; however, in the presence of a neurological injury a more thorough evaluation is necessary. Bedrest and symptomatic relief is the initial therapeutic regimen.

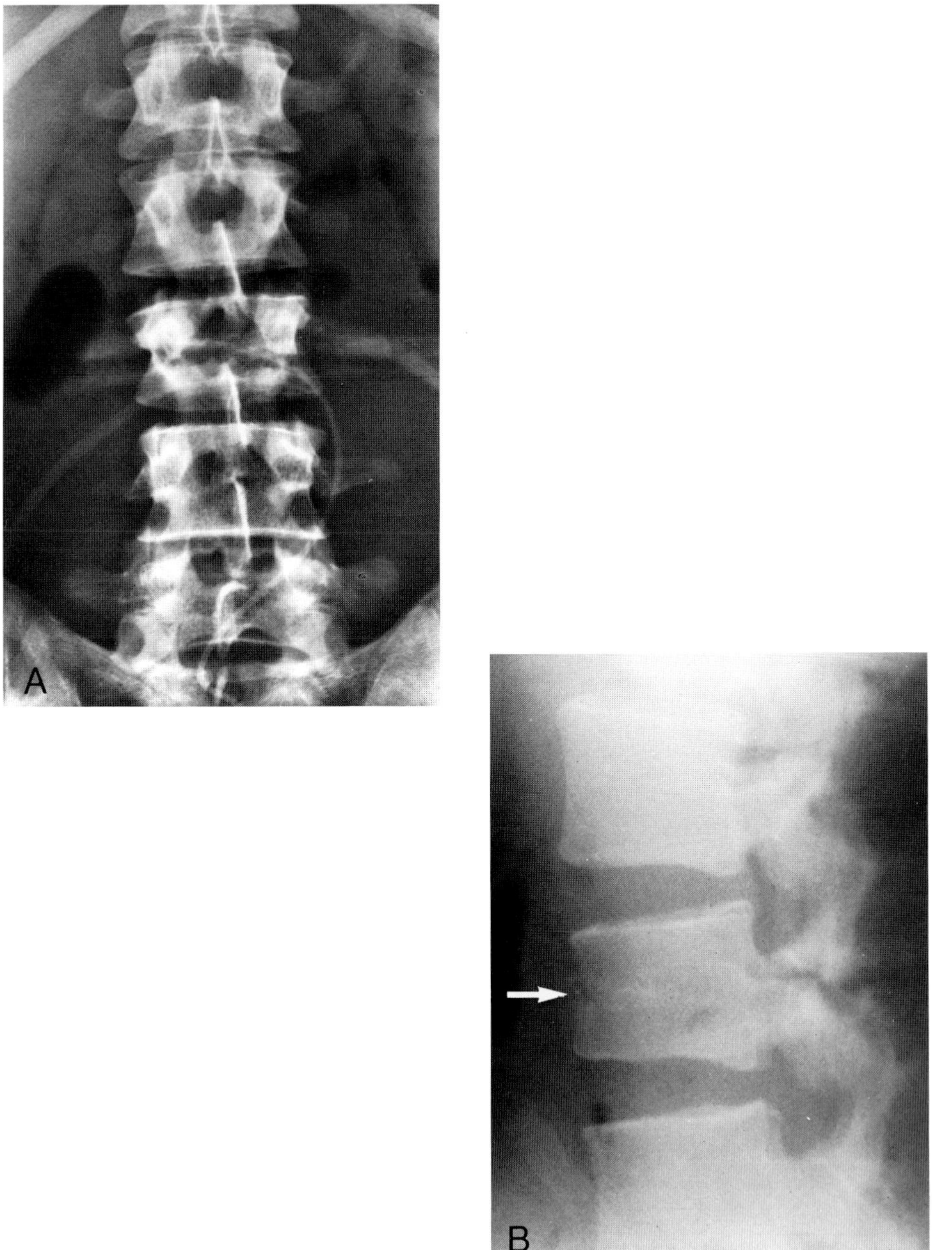

Fig. 3-7. Chance fracture of L3. (A) AP view. Note the ovoid appearance of the spinous process of L3. (B) The lateral view demonstrates the fracture line running through the vertebral body and the posterior elements.

Spondylolisthesis

Spondylolisthesis (Fig. 3-8) is the subluxation of one vertebral body on the one below it. There may be a variety of reasons for this occurrence. One specific etiology is isthmic or spondylolytic spondylolisthesis; this is due to a defect in the pars interarticularis. This condition is usually chronic and can be differentiated from an acute fracture by examining the edges of the defect. In an acute injury, the edge is rough and irregular in comparison to the smooth, well-rounded contour of the chronic condition. If differentiation cannot be made via roentgenograms, a technetium bone scan will give definitive information.

CLINICAL PRESENTATION

Back pain is the most common presentation. Neurological deficit is rare.

ROENTGENOGRAMS

AP, lateral, and oblique roentgenograms with a "spot" lateral of L5-S1 should be obtained. The oblique view (Fig. 3-9) is best to see the defect in the pars intra-articularis and the "Scotty dog." The most frequent level for isthmic spondylolisthesis is L5-S1.

COMPLICATIONS

Acute neurological deficit is rare. Discogenic disease at the level above the spondylolisthesis has increased incidence.

TREATMENT

Symptomatic relief with bedrest and analgesics. Chronic isthmic spondylolisthesis may require surgery if symptoms warrant.

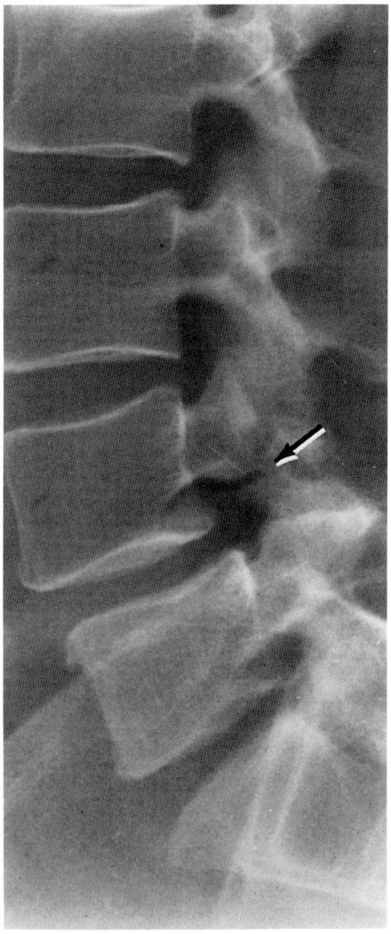

Fig. 3-8. Spondylolisthesis of L4 on L5. This is less common than that seen at L5-S1.

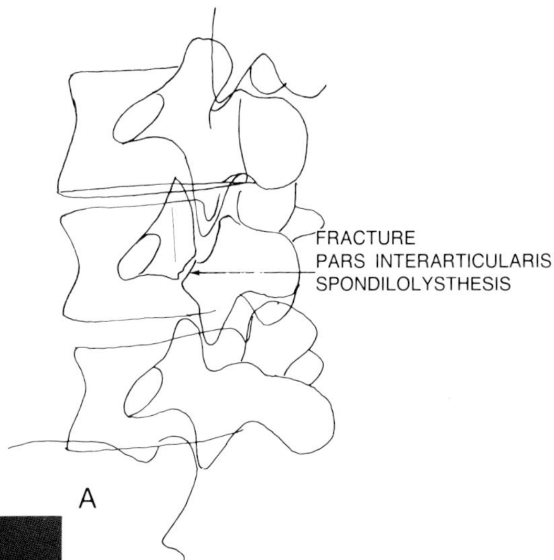

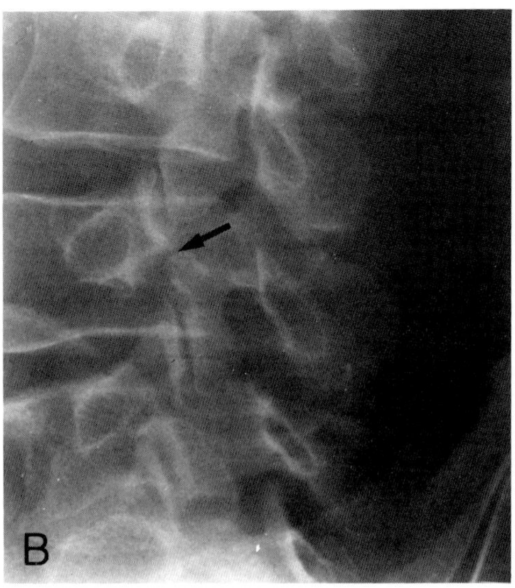

Fig. 3-9. Spondylolisthesis. (A) One can see the defect in the pars interarticularis on the lateral view (arrow). (B) The oblique view delineates the "scotty dog" and more clearly shows the pars defect as a collar or a broken neck on the scotty dog (arrow).

Lumbosacral Strain (Low Back Pain) and Herniated Nucleus Pulposus

This is the most common low back problem. The patient complains of low back pain without radiation, muscle spasm, decreased motion, and tenderness. Severity of pain is variable, but the patient may be unable to walk. Hospitalization may be needed for the patient who cannot ambulate, but the patient can usually be managed with bedrest at home. Roentgenograms are normal. Bedrest is the most important treatment. The addition of mild analgesics and moist heat will add to the patient's comfort. The role of anti-inflammatory medications and muscle relaxants is controversial.

With herniated nucleus pulposus (ruptured disc), patients give the same history as those with lumbosacral strain. However, the former usually complain of leg pain (below the knee) and/or numbness and may also have muscle weakness, specific for the nerve root involved. The plain roentgenograms are normal. These patients may have lost a deep tendon reflex, may have a positive straight-leg raising test, and may have increasing pain in the leg upon coughing or sneezing. The initial management of these patients is identical to those with lumbosacral strain, but the addition of anti-inflammatory medication for these patients is well supported. Follow-up care is essential for patients with radicular pain.

PART II

The Upper Extremities

Larry S. Eisenfeld
Robert J. Neviaser

4
The Shoulder and Humerus

SHOULDER

The shoulder is the most mobile joint in the body. As a result, it is also susceptible to a wide variety of injuries. Since the joint involves three bones—the clavicle, the scapula and the humerus—an injury to any one can affect shoulder function. We will consider each bone individually, as well as the dislocations associated with their articulations. Routine radiographs are AP (Fig. 4-1A), axillary (Fig. 4-1B), or tangential "Y" (Fig. 4-1C) or transthoracic (Fig. 4-1D) views.

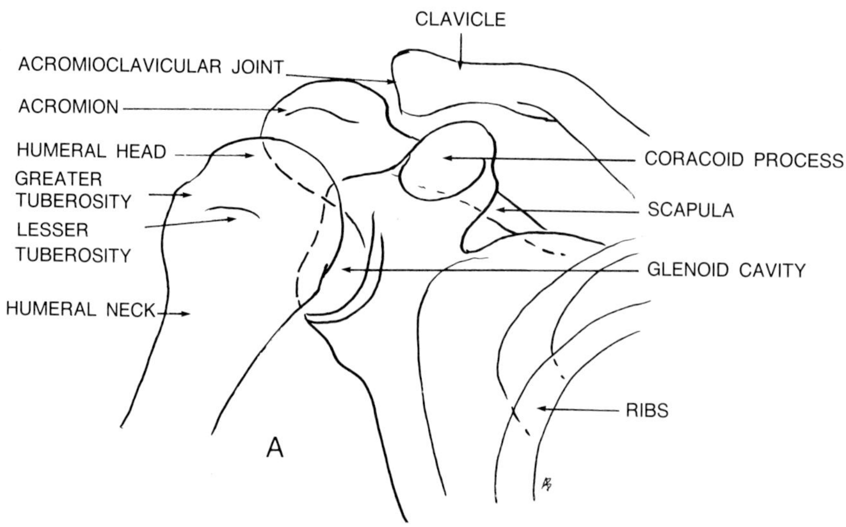

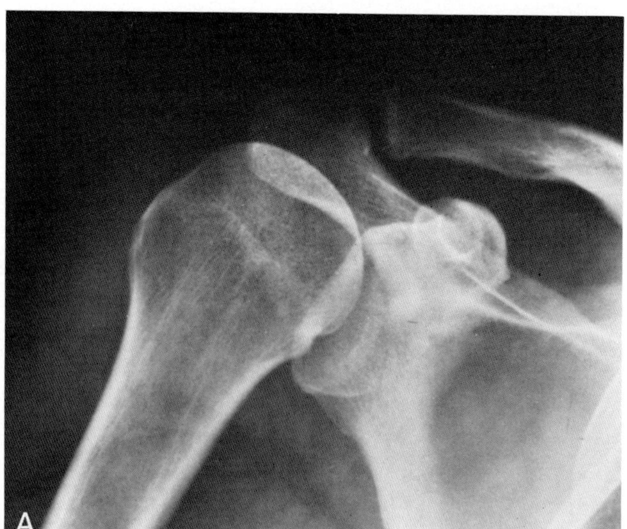

Fig. 4-1. (A) (Figure continues).

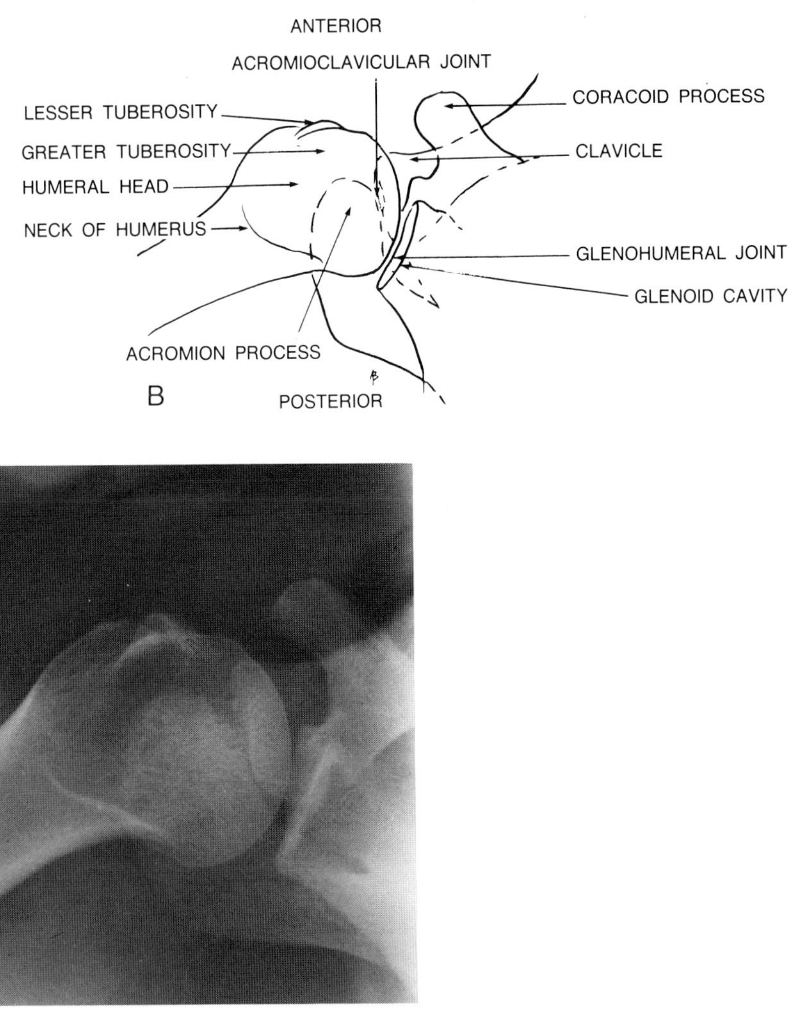

Fig. 4-1. (A) AP of the shoulder — normal. (B) Axillary view of the shoulder — normal. The coracoid process defines the anterior aspect of the shoulder joint (Figure continues).

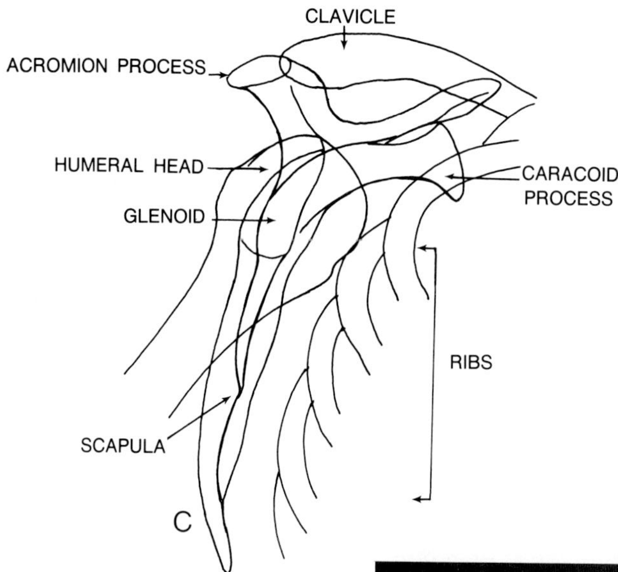

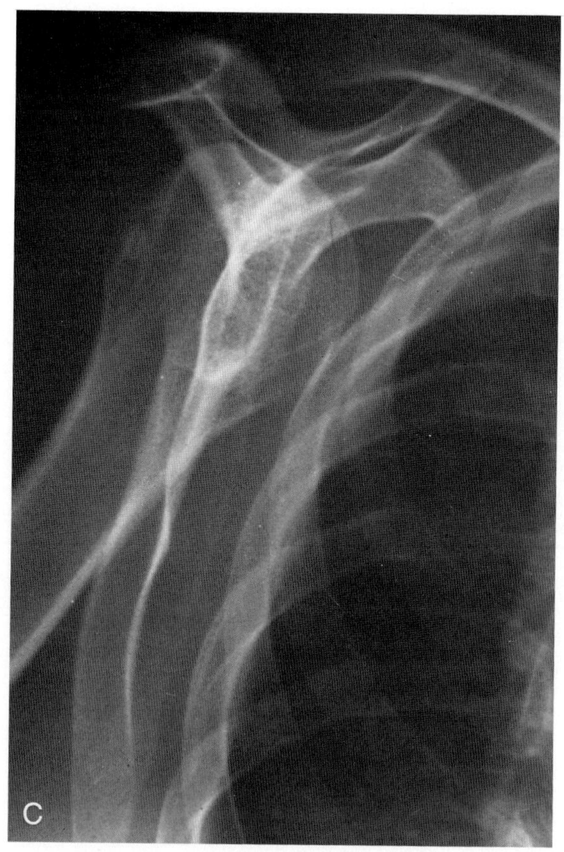

Fig. 4-1. (C) (Figure continues).

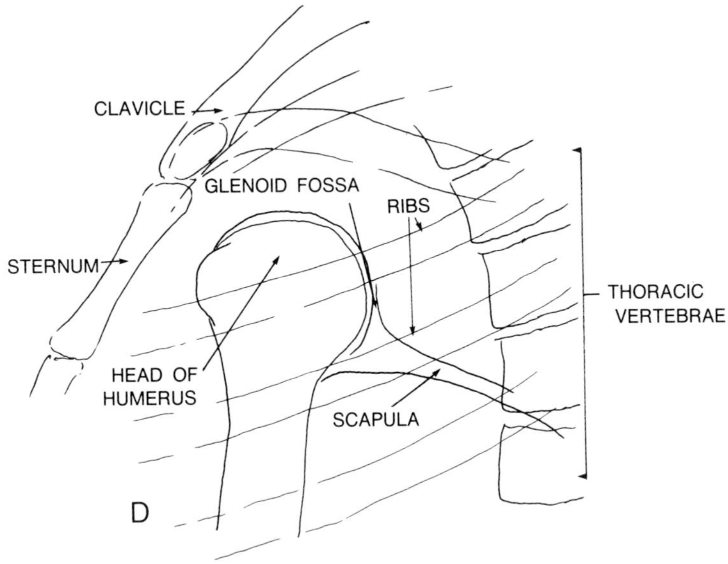

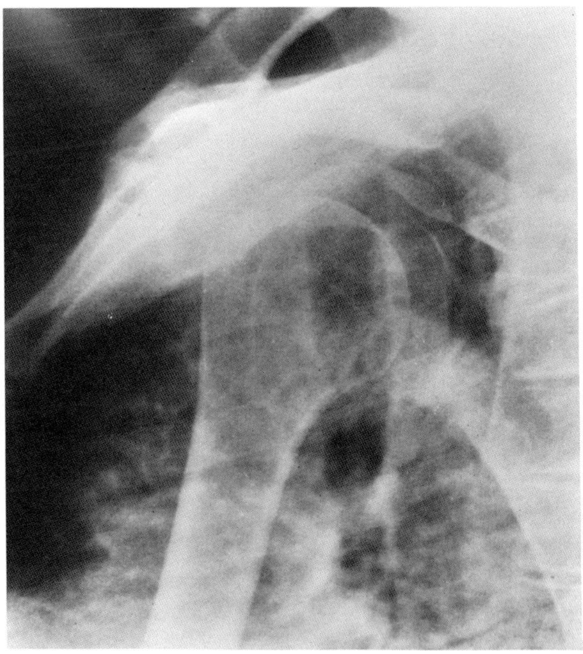

Fig. 4-1 (continued). (C) Tangential "Y" view of the scapula. The humeral head is centered in the vertex of the "Y" formed by the coracoid process on one side and the spine of the scapula on the other side. The other limb of the "Y" formed by the body of the scapula. (D) Transthoracic (trauma) lateral. This reveals the location of the humeral head, but is poor to visualize detail of fractures.

Fractures of the Clavicle

Fractures of the clavicle are common, especially in children.

MECHANISM

An indirect lateral or posterolateral force usually produces fractures at the proximal or middle third. A fall in which the shoulder is struck from above produces a fracture of the distal third, or an acromioclavicular injury.

CLINICAL PRESENTATION

The patient has localized tenderness at the site of the injury. The arm is held against the chest and any motion is resisted. Most fractures (80 percent) are in the middle third, 15 percent are in the distal third, and 5 percent are in the proximal third.

ROENTGENOGRAMS

An AP view of the clavicle (Fig. 4-2) and an apical lordotic view (45° cephalad) are recommended for maximum detail. The glenohumeral joint must be visualized on at least one roentgenogram to rule out an associated dislocation.

COMPLICATIONS

Complications are uncommon but neurovascular injury can occur. Nonunion is rare. Malunion is common, although not often disabling.

TREATMENT

A figure-of-eight clavicular strap is appropriate treatment for proximal or middle third fractures. For fractures of the distal third, a sling may suffice, but if it is displaced, open reduction and internal fixation may be required.

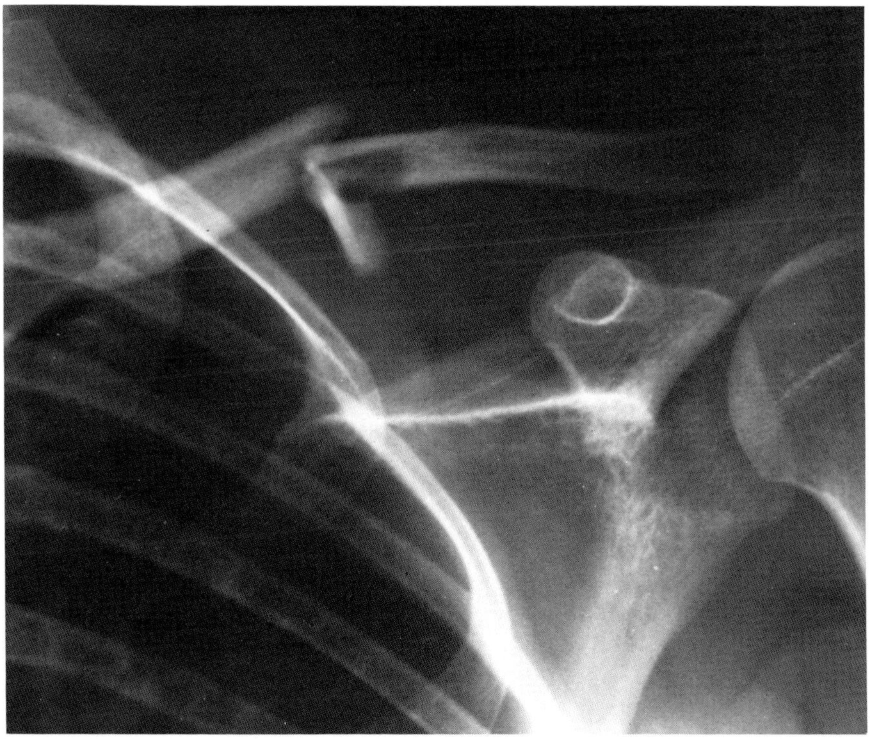

Fig. 4-2. Clavicle fracture — mid shaft.

Fractures of the Scapula

Scapular fractures are rare.

MECHANISM

This fracture results from a direct force applied to the scapula. Since the forces necessary to produce this fracture are great, associated life-threatening injuries to the chest, vertebrae, and blood vessels can occur.

CLINICAL PRESENTATION

The patient holds the arm at the side and resists any motion of the arm or the shoulder. There is diffuse swelling and tenderness over the scapula.

ROENTGENOGRAMS

Since this injury presents in a similar fashion to a shoulder injury, the initial roengtgenograms (Fig. 4-3) obtained are usually that of the shoulder. In addition to these films, a true lateral of the scapula should be obtained.

COMPLICATIONS

Any associated injuries to the chest, spine, and blood vessels are of primary importance.

TREATMENT

Symptomatic relief, accomplished by immobilization with a sling and swathe for control of motion of the arm is recommended.

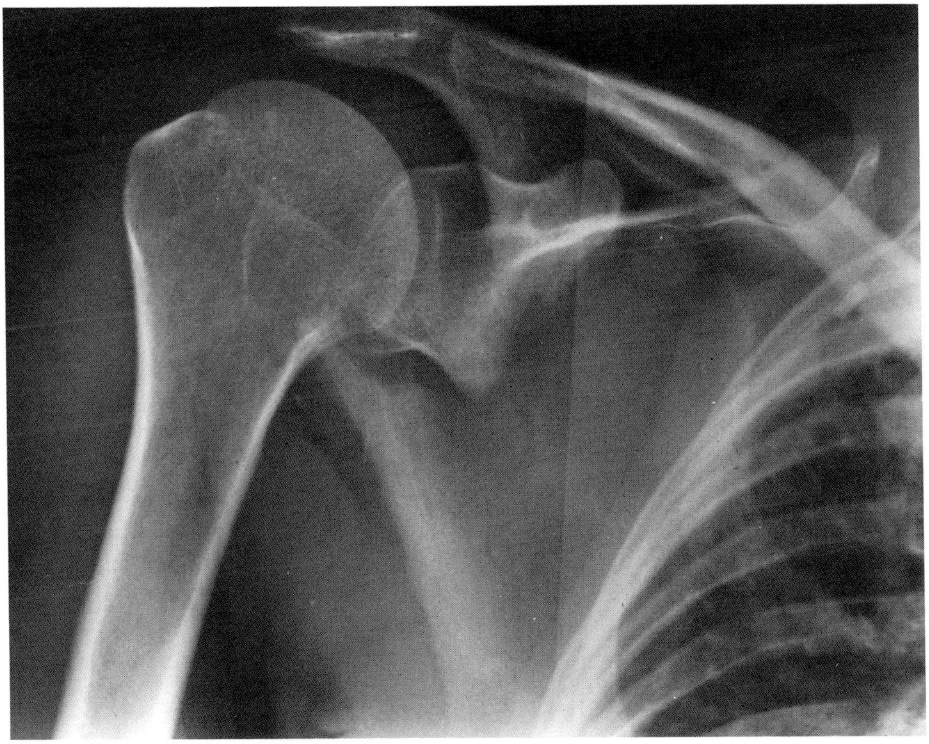

Fig. 4-3. Scapula fracture — neck of the scapula.

Acromioclavicular Dislocation (Shoulder Separation)

MECHANISM

A fall on the acromion or superolateral aspect of the shoulder.

CLINICAL PRESENTATION

Pain and swelling are localized at the acromioclavicular joint (A/C). The distal end of the clavicle may be prominent and "free-floating."

ROENTGENOGRAMS

An AP view of the shoulder or specifically of the acromioclavicular joint should be obtained. A comparison view of the opposite side is useful and weights may be hung from each hand to help determine the extent of the injury. The patient should be erect with the arm hanging free when the roentgenograms are taken. These injuries are classified into three grades. A Grade I injury shows no subluxation of the clavicle, but there may be an increased width between the acromion and the clavicle. A Grade II injury shows the lateral aspect of the clavicle to be subluxed superiorly but still in some contact with the acromion. A Grade III injury shows the lateral clavicle to be dislocated from the acromion (Fig. 4-4).

COMPLICATIONS

There also may be a fracture of the clavicle, the coracoid process, or acromion. The main complication is ossification of the trapezoid and coronoid ligaments, which may occur in 50 percent of patients.

TREATMENT

Analgesics are given for symptomatic relief. Grade I and Grade II injuries may be treated with a sling. Some Grade II and Grade III injuries may require late reconstruction, if disabling.

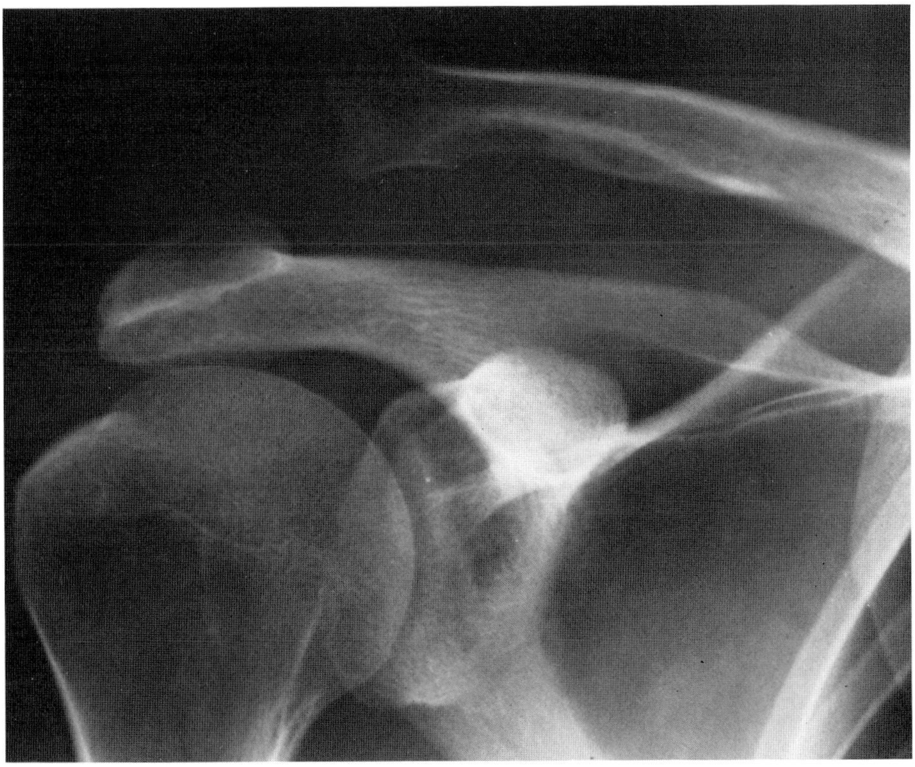

Fig. 4-4. Acromioclavicular separation. The complete separation between the clavicle and the acromion represents a third degree separation.

Sternoclavicular Dislocation

MECHANISM

This injury results from a great force, usually due to vehicular accidents (80%) or sports (20%). Anterior dislocation is most common and is the result of a force to the anterior surface of the shoulder which is transmitted along the clavicle and dislocates it anterior to the sternum. The rarer posterior dislocation is from a direct blow to the anteromedial portion of the clavicle, forcing it posteriorly.

CLINICAL PRESENTATION

There is either an increased or decreased prominence of the medial aspect of the clavicle, depending on the direction of the dislocation. Posterior dislocation is much more serious and may produce venous congestion, shortness of breath, diminished circulation to the ipsilateral arm, dysphagia, pneumothorax, or compression of mediastinal structures.

ROENTGENOGRAMS

An AP view of the clavicle or a chest roentgenogram usually confirms the diagnosis. However, correlation with the clinical situation is helpful. Tomography or computerized tomography may be necessary for additional information. A chest roentgenogram should be taken to exclude pneumothorax.

COMPLICATIONS

Complications are rare with anterior dislocations, but may be life-threatening with a posterior dislocation.

TREATMENT

Closed reduction as soon as possible, often requiring general anesthesia.

SHOULDER DISLOCATIONS

The shoulder (glenohumeral joint) is the most commonly dislocated major joint. Eighty-five percent of these are anterior dislocations.

Anterior Dislocation

MECHANISM

Forced abduction, external rotation, and extension of the shoulder are responsible for this injury.

CLINICAL PRESENTATION

Severe pain is present. The affected arm is held in slight abduction and supported by the opposite hand. The acromion is prominent and the normal contour of the shoulder is lost. The coracoid is less prominent, and the humeral head may be palpable anteriorly. Any motion is painful, especially external rotation. Anterior dislocations are divided into subcoracoid, subglenoid, and the rare injuries of subclavicular and intrathoracic dislocations.

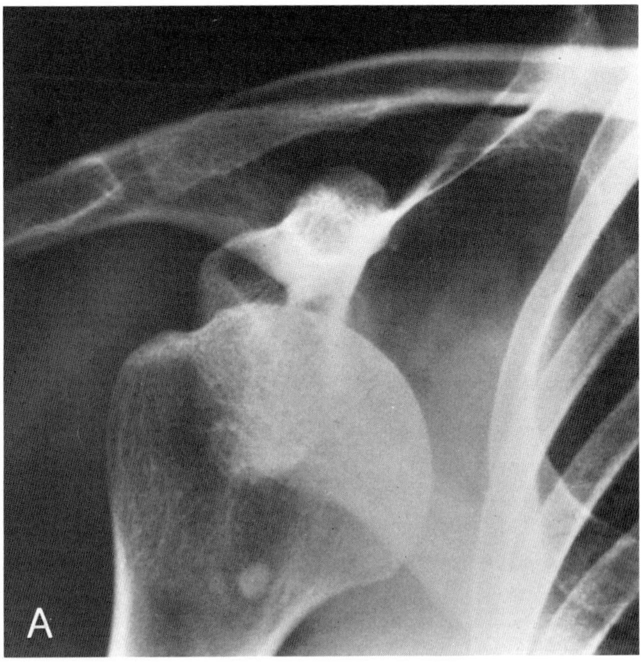

Fig. 4-5. Anterior dislocation of the shoulder. (A) AP view. Note that the head of the humerus is anterior and inferior to the corocoid process.

ROENTGENOGRAMS

An AP view of the shoulder shows that the humeral head is not in apposition to the glenoid (Fig. 4-5A). A transthoracic view (trauma lateral view) (Fig. 4-5B) can reveal whether the head is anterior or posterior to the glenoid cavity, but it is often extremely difficult to interpret. The axillary view (Fig. 4-5C) is the optimal view for defining the relationship of the humeral head to the glenoid, as well as whether or not a fracture is present. It may be uncomfortable to position the patient to obtain the axillary view, but if necessary, analgesics may be given prior to taking the roentgenograms. Usually patience and gentle positioning of the arm to 30 degrees of abduction is technically sufficient for this view. The axillary view is vastly superior to the transthoracic view or the tangential view of the scapula.

COMPLICATIONS

Axillary nerve, artery or vein injury, brachial plexus injury, rotator cuff tears (especially in patients over 40), and associated fractures of the coracoid process, glenoid and/or greater tuberosity are the most common injuries. Young patients may be subject to recurrent dislocations.

TREATMENT

Reduction as soon as possible and immobilization in sling and swathe.

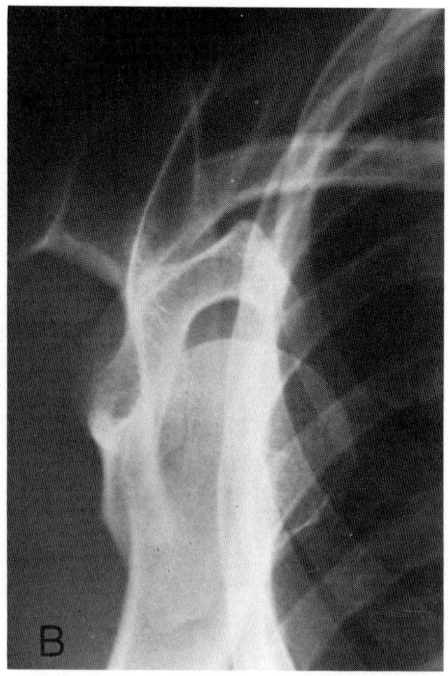

Fig. 4-5. (B) (Figure continues).

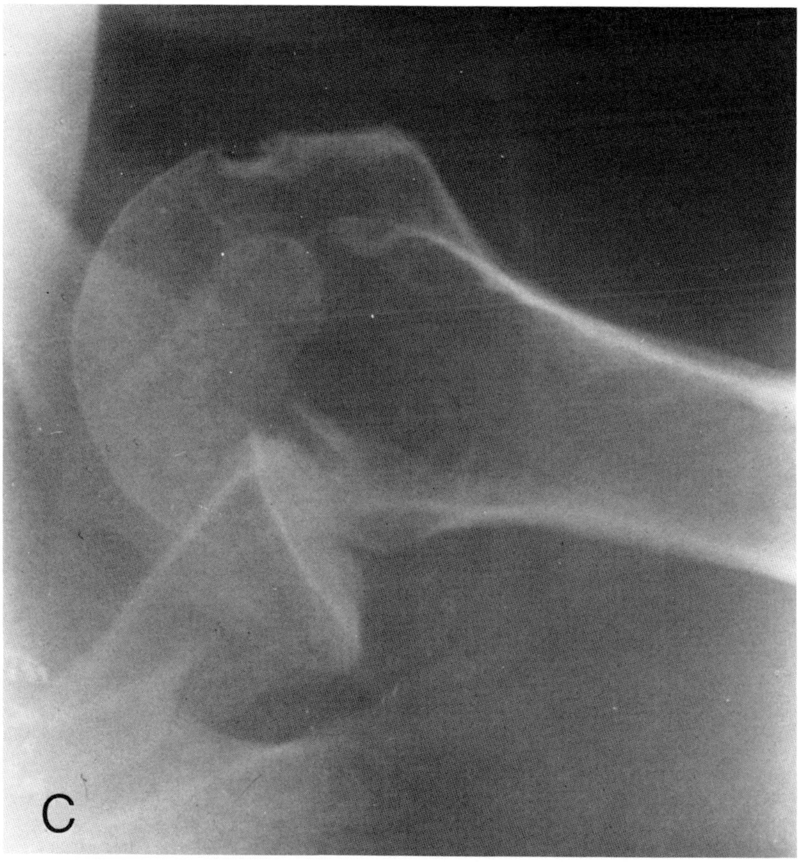

Fig. 4-5 (continued). (B) "Y" view. (C) Axillary view. The humeral head does not articulate with the glenoid but is superimposed on the corocoid process (anterior).

Posterior Dislocation

This is the *most commonly missed* major dislocation in the body.

MECHANISM

The highest incidence of posterior dislocations of the shoulder occurs with the patient having a seizure. The dislocation occurs with the shoulder flexed, adducted, and internally rotated.

CLINICAL PRESENTATION

The arm is held tightly against the chest in internal rotation and adduction. The coracoid process is unusually prominent and the usual contour of the shoulder is distorted. The arm is fixed in internal rotation and cannot be rotated externally.

ROENTGENOGRAMS

The AP view reveals an "ice cream cone" appearance of the humeral head and the loss of the elliptical overlap of the head and glenoid (Fig. 4-6A). A distance greater than 6 mm between the anterior glenoid and humeral head is highly

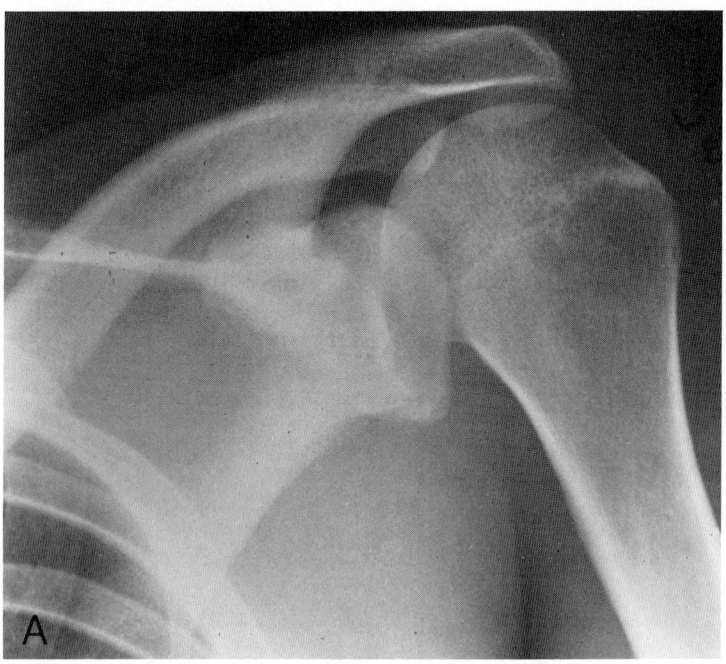

suggestive of posterior dislocation. The *axillary view* (Fig. 4-6B) is the most important view for making the diagnosis. Posterior dislocations are *missed at least 50 percent of the time* without an axillary view. The humeral head is seen to be displaced posterior to the glenoid.

COMPLICATIONS

Missing the diagnosis is the major problem. Fractures of the humeral head or shaft, especially of the lesser tuberosity, occur in virtually all patients with this dislocation. Neurovascular injuries are rare.

TREATMENT

Reduction as soon as possible and immobilization in a sling and swathe is indicated.

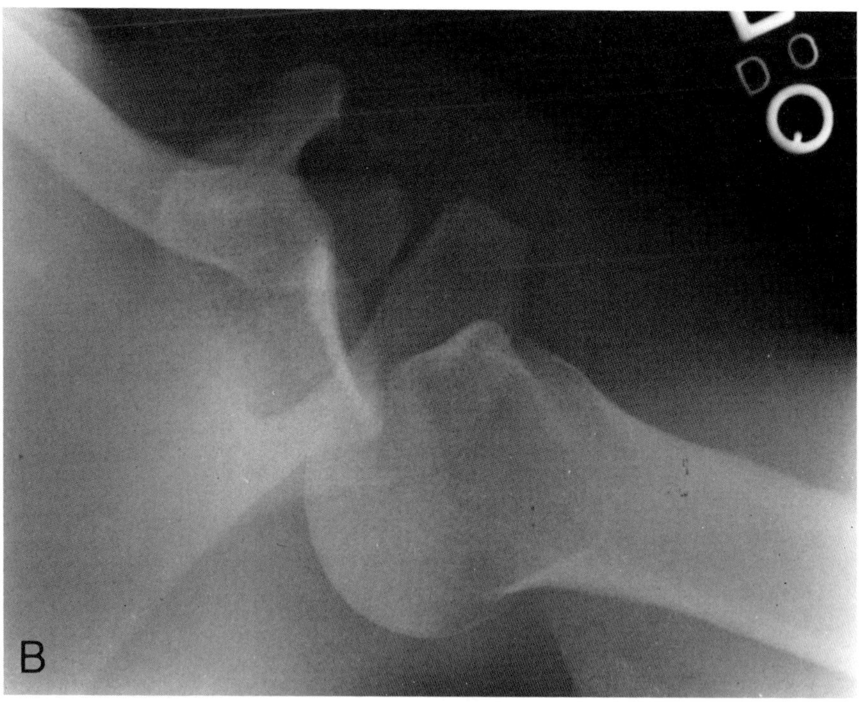

Fig. 4-6. Posterior dislocation of the shoulder. (A) AP view reveals the "ice cream cone" appearance of the humeral head as well as the elliptical overlap of the humeral head on the glenoid. (B) Axillary view clearly shows the humeral head to be posterior to the glenoid.

Fracture — Dislocations

MECHANISM

The same mechanics that produce the routine dislocation are involved, but there is usually greater force involved in the fracture-dislocation.

CLINICAL PRESENTATION

The presentation is identical to that of routine dislocations; however, swelling and ecchymosis are also present.

ROENTGENOGRAMS

There are classically four areas of the upper humerus: the greater tuberosity, the lesser tuberosity, the humeral head, and the shaft. An important reason for obtaining a pre-reduction roentgenogram of a shoulder dislocation is to determine if any associated fracture exists. It is important to have a good axillary view as well as an AP roentgenogram to define the number of fragments and the extent of their displacement (Fig. 4-7).

COMPLICATIONS

A fracture dislocation may not be reducible with closed methods. The greater the number of fragments involving the head and tuberosities, the greater the likelihood of closed reduction being unsuccessful. If so, open reduction and internal fixation may be needed. Aseptic necrosis of the humeral head may occur. Rotator cuff tears occur with any fracture of the greater tuberosity, but can heal if their fracture is anatomically reduced. Malunion is high with inadequate reduction or treatment.

TREATMENT

Closed or open reduction of the dislocation, depending on the nature of the particular injury.

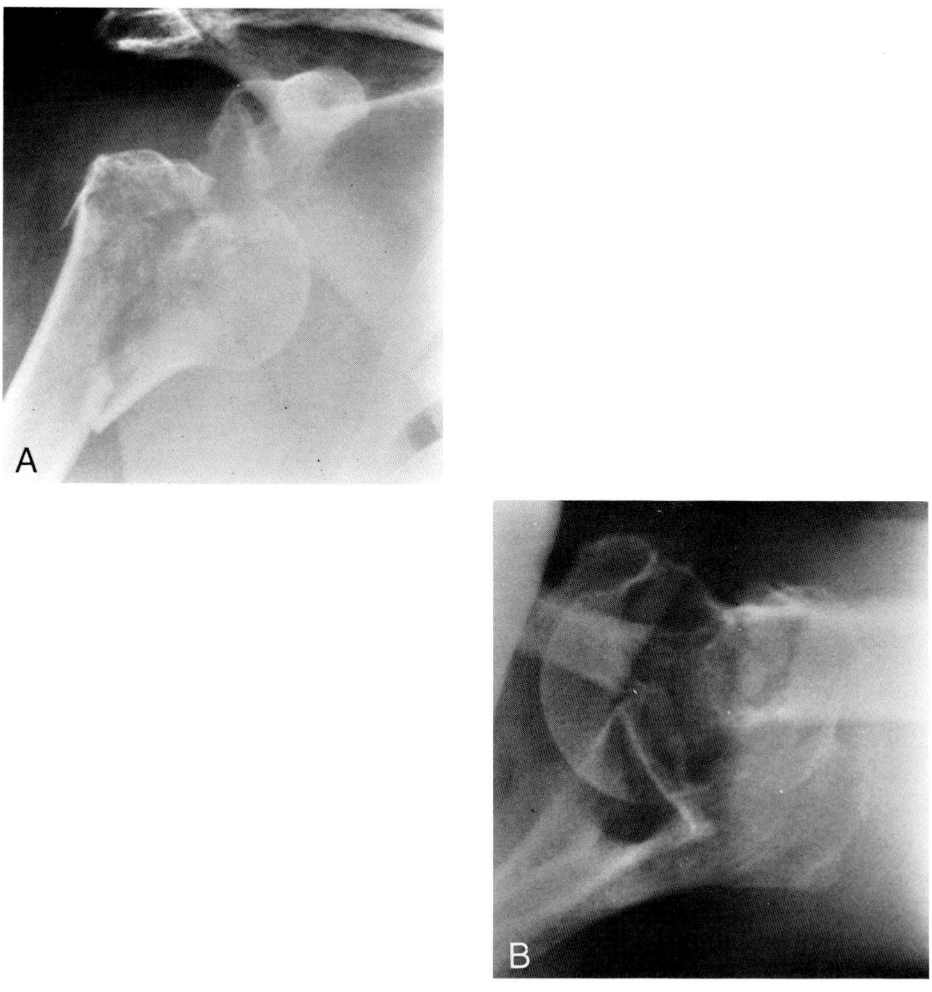

Fig. 4-7. Fracture dislocation of the shoulder. (A) AP view shows the subglenoid position of the humeral head. (B) Axillary view.

HUMERUS

Fractures of the humerus are separated into three categories: proximal, shaft, and supracondylar. Routine radiographs are the AP (Fig. 4-8A) and lateral views (Fig. 4-8B), which should include the shoulder joint as well as the elbow joint. Supracondylar fractures will be discussed in Chapter 5, The Elbow.

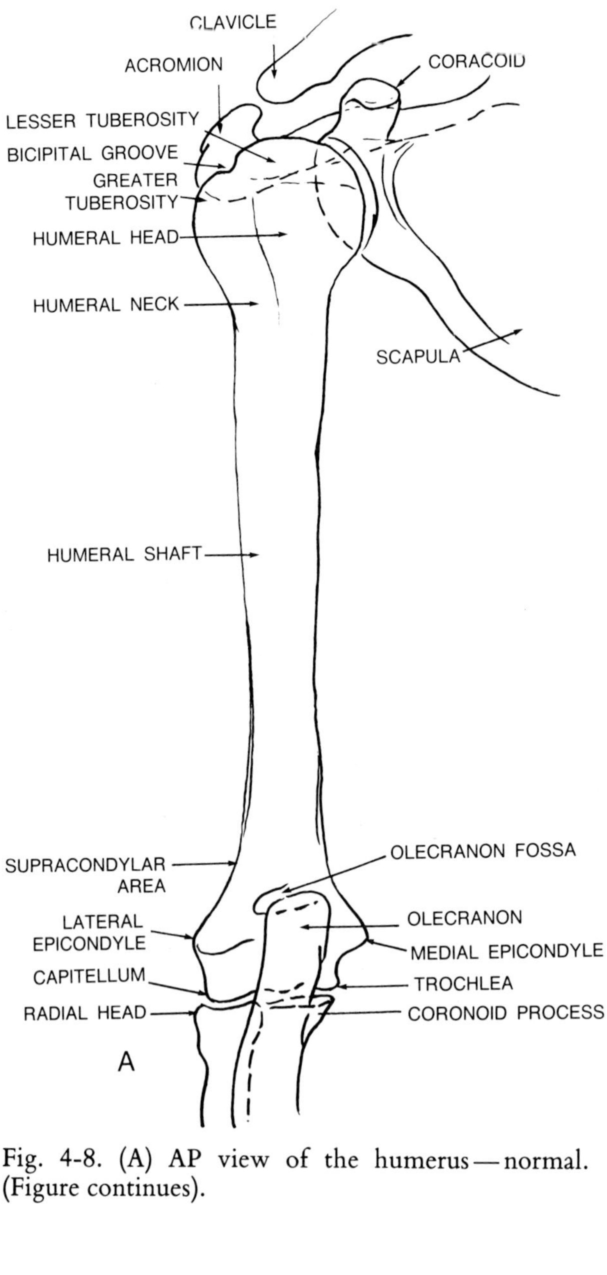

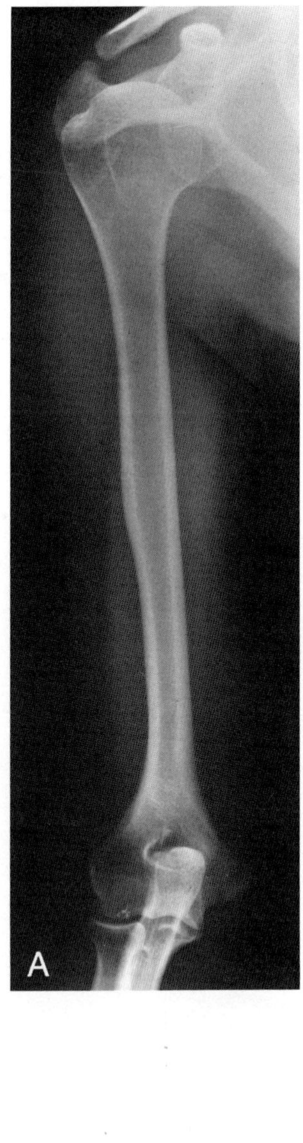

Fig. 4-8. (A) AP view of the humerus—normal. (Figure continues).

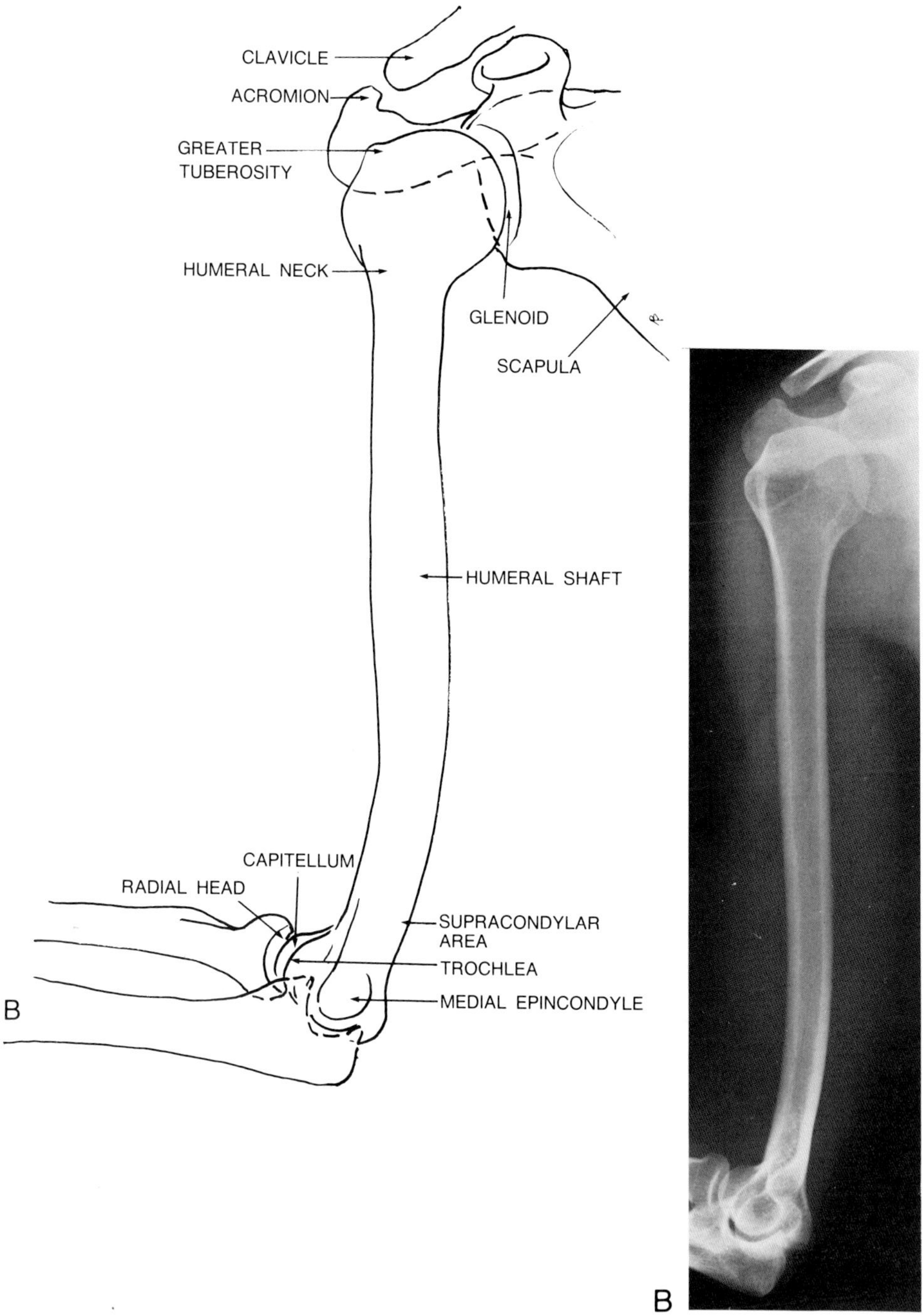

Fig. 4-8 (Continued). (B) Lateral view of the humerus — normal.

Fractures of the Proximal Humerus

This includes fractures of the head, greater tuberosity, lesser tuberosity and neck. Eighty percent are minimally displaced.

MECHANISM

A fall on the outstretched arm or a direct blow to the proximal humerus produces this injury.

CLINICAL PRESENTATION

Marked swelling and tenderness exist. Crepitus may be present with or without motion of the arm. Motion is restricted by pain.

ROENTGENOGRAMS

AP and axillary views (Fig. 4-9) should be obtained in all cases. Again, it may take more time and effort to obtain the axillary view, but since it provides the most useful information, the effort is justified. Adequate roentgenograms are essential to evaluate the injury fully, especially for displacement of the fragment. If the lesser tuberosity is fractured, one must be sure to rule out a posterior dislocation. Humeral neck fractures (Fig. 4-10) are quite common in the elderly.

COMPLICATIONS

Nerve injuries, which are rare, are usually confined to the axillary nerve. Calcific deposits may be confused with a fracture. Malunion, stiffness, and aseptic necrosis of the humeral head may also occur.

TREATMENT

The principles of reduction are as previously discussed for fracture dislocations. Greater tuberosity fractures need open reduction and internal fixation if displaced. Associated rotator cuff tears occur with this injury and should be repaired if open reduction is carried out. Lesser tuberosity fractures can be treated with sling and swathe even if displaced. Closed reduction of head and neck fractures into acceptable alignment may be achieved. Comminuted fractures of the head can result in aseptic necrosis. If closed reduction cannot be achieved, open reduction should be undertaken.

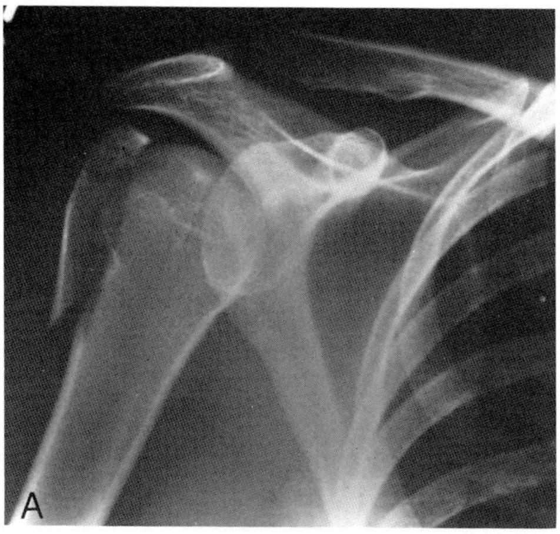

Fig. 4-9. Greater tuberosity fracture. (A) AP view. (B) Axillary view demonstrates the significant displacement of this fracture.

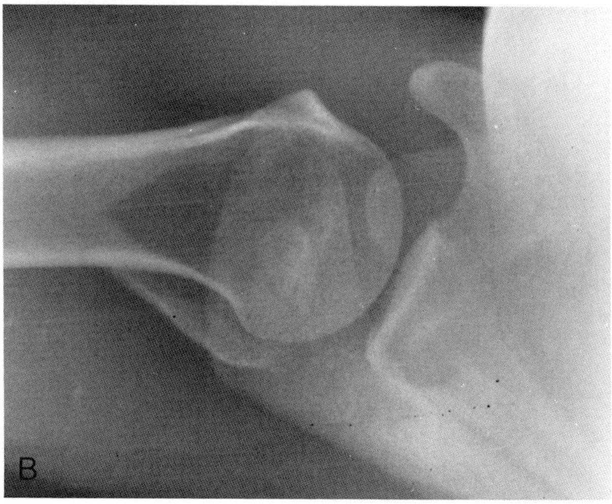

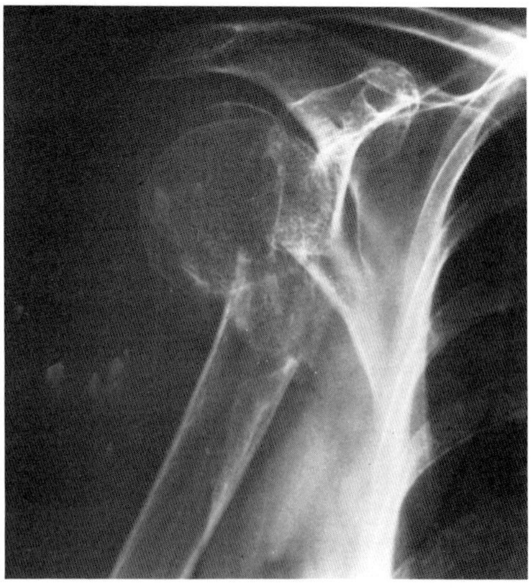

Fig. 4-10. Fracture of the surgical neck of the humerus.

Humeral Shaft Fractures

MECHANISM

An indirect injury from a fall on the elbow or outstretched arm is the primary mechanism of injury. A direct blow to the arm can also produce humeral shaft fractures.

CLINICAL PRESENTATION

The arm may appear shortened, grossly swollen, and deformed. Crepitus and abnormal motion can be present. A baseline initial neurovascular examination should be done with specific reference to the radial nerve.

ROENTGENOGRAMS

AP and lateral roentgenograms (Fig. 4-11) are necessary, but the examination should include the shoulder and elbow joints. The fracture can be spiral, transverse, or comminuted, depending on the mechanism of injury.

COMPLICATIONS

Radial nerve injury (5 – 10%) can present as a wrist drop. It is usually a neuropraxia, and early exploration of the nerve is not necessary except in open fractures. Vascular injuries are emergencies, but are rare. Evaluation of the fracture for pathological etiology may be indicated as this is a common place for metastasis.

TREATMENT

Sling and swathe is satisfactory temporary immobilization. The final choice of treatment modality is quite variable, depending on the fracture and the treating surgeon.

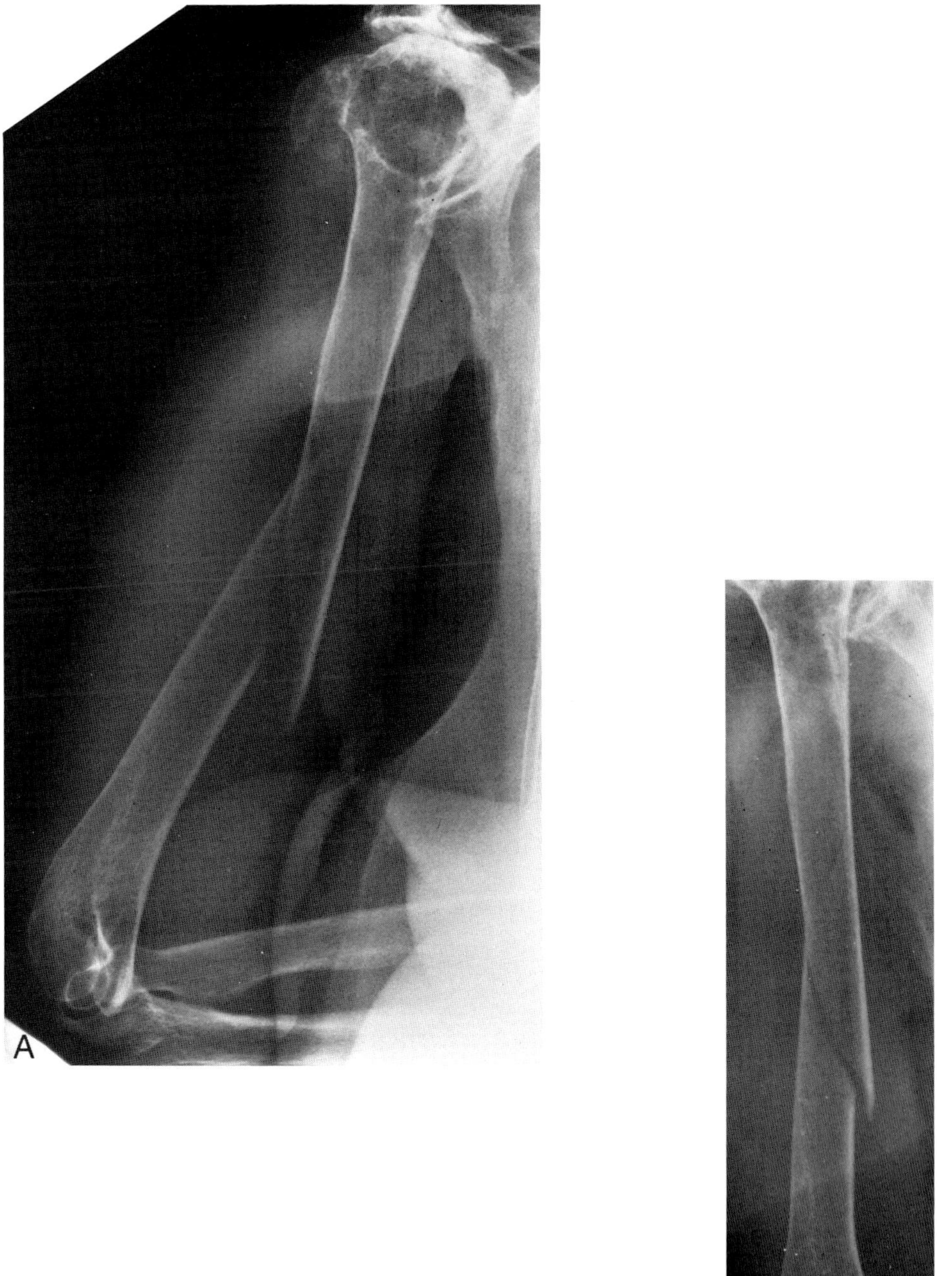

Fig. 4-11. Humeral shaft fracture. (A) AP view. The course of the radial nerve along the humerus should always be remembered. (B) Lateral view.

5
The Elbow

Six percent of all fractures occur in and around the elbow. Routine radiographs require an AP (Fig. 5-1C) and lateral view (Fig. 5-1A) as a minimum; with additional information often gained on the oblique view (Fig. 5-1B). The elbow joint has three articulations: humero-ulnar, humero-radial and radioulnar. There is a normal valgus inclination, the "carrying angle," of 5 to 20 degrees (average 15 degrees), of the elbow. The normal anatomic relationships

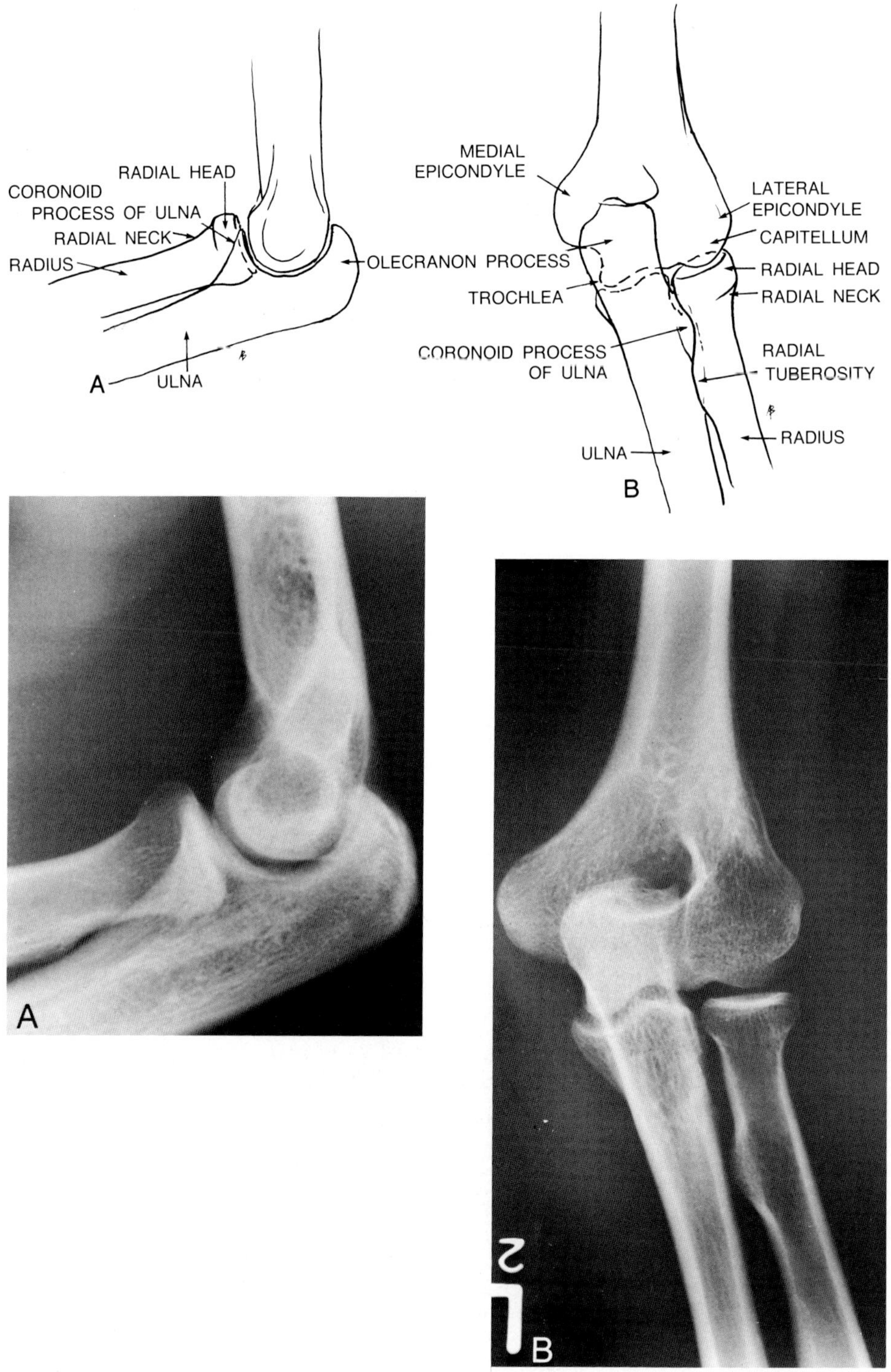

Fig. 5-1. (A) Lateral view of the elbow—normal. (B) Oblique view of the elbow—normal.

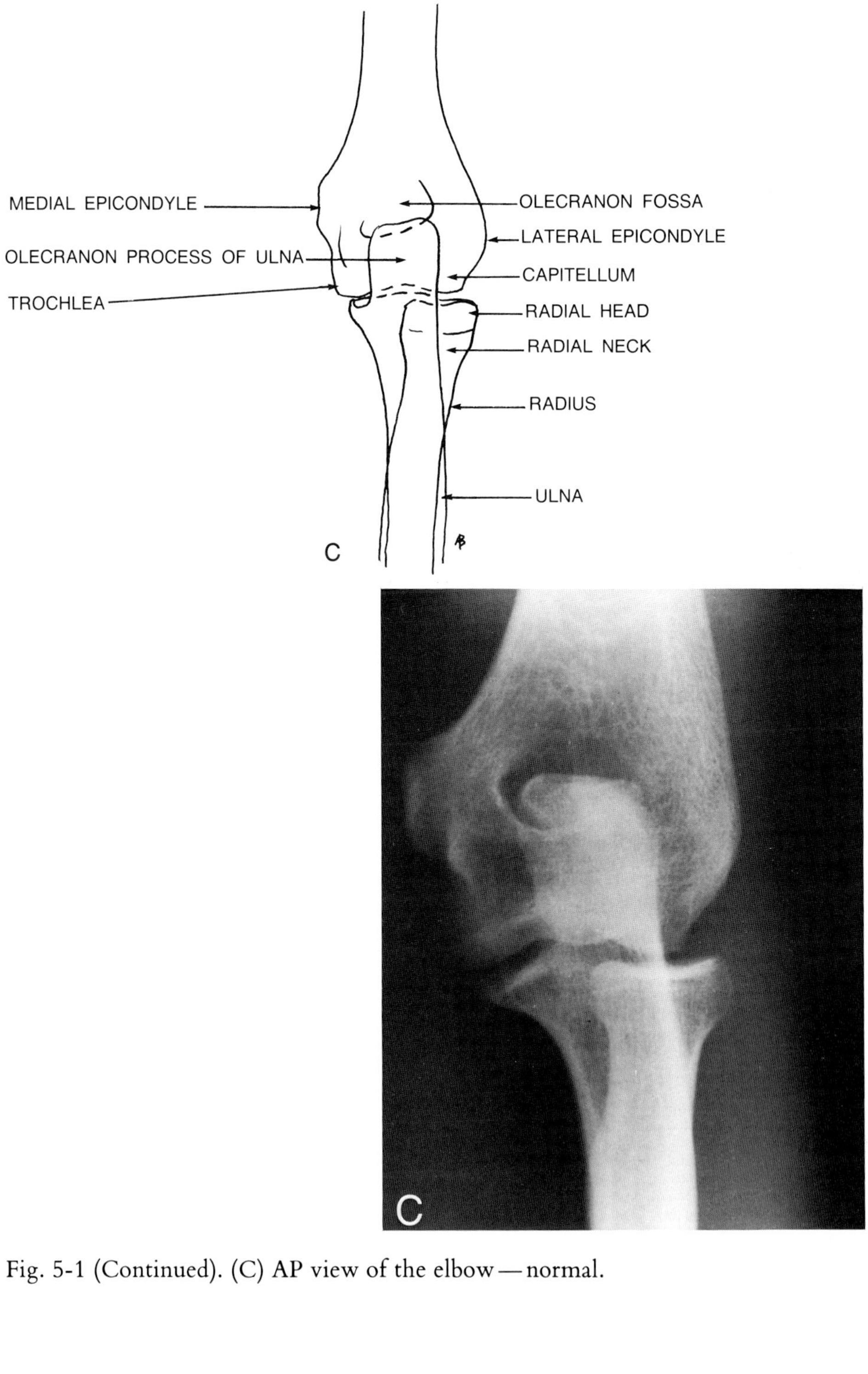

Fig. 5-1 (Continued). (C) AP view of the elbow — normal.

in the elbow include: (1) a straight line drawn on the anterior radial shaft should pass through the capitellum in all radiographic views (Fig. 5-2); and (2) an equilateral triangle is formed by the olecranon, the medial, and the lateral epicondyle (Fig. 5-3). When there is a dislocation, the above relationships are disrupted. Fractures about the elbow include those of the supracondylar region of the humerus, humeral condyles, the capitellum, the trochlea, the olecranon, and the radial head. Any fracture of the articular surface results in hemarthrosis, which will elevate the anterior and/or the posterior fat pad, producing the roentgenographic "fat pad sign" (Fig. 5-4).

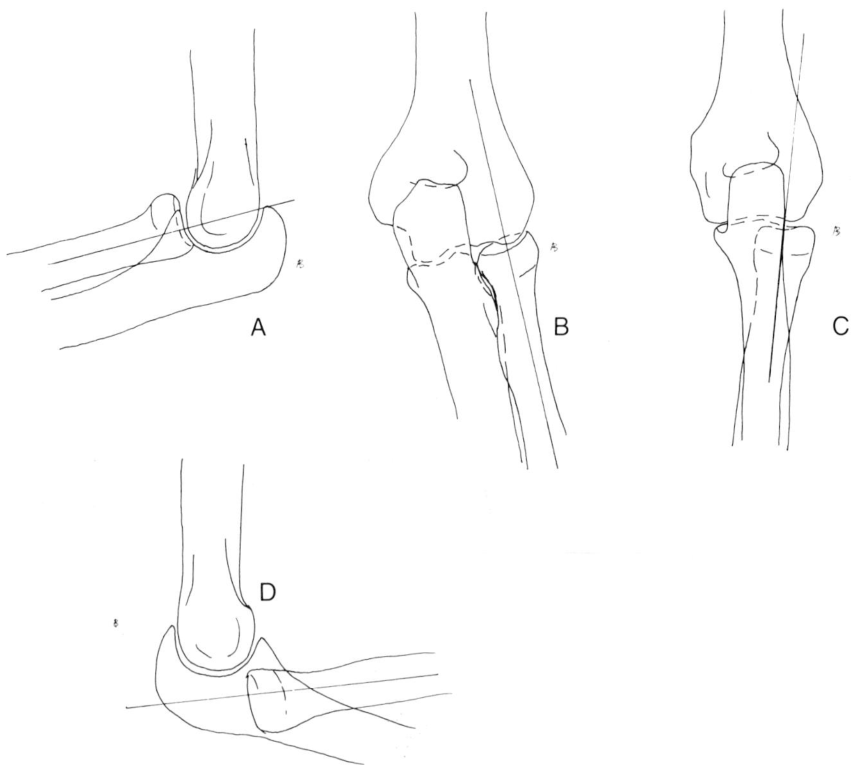

Fig. 5-2. Radial capitellar alignment. A line through the shaft of the radius on any view should intersect the capitellum if the radius is located. Note that part D reveals the loss of this relationship with a radial head dislocation.

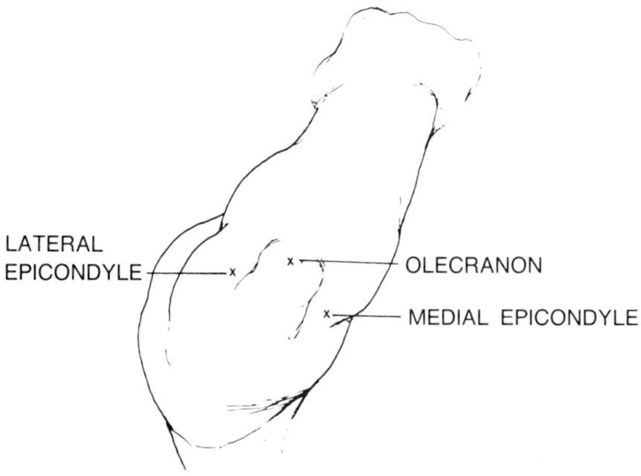

Fig. 5-3. The equilateral triangle. In the normal elbow, an equilateral triangle is formed between the medial and lateral epicondyles and the olecranon process.

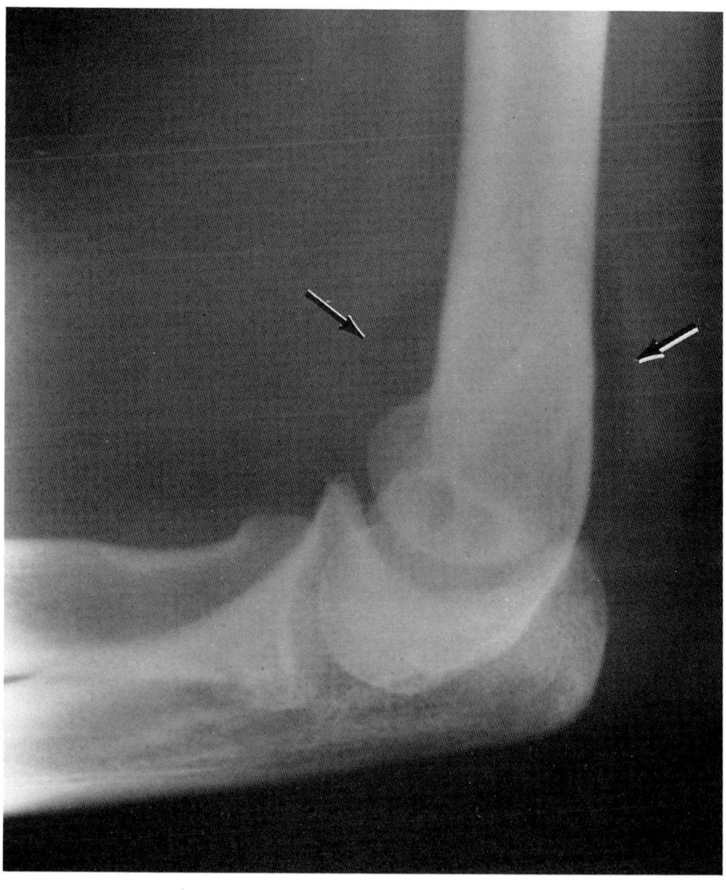

Fig. 5-4. "Fat pad" sign. This is indicative of fluid within the joint. This is usually blood representing an intra-articular injury. If no other fracture is seen, this most often represents a radial head fracture.

Supracondylar Fractures of the Humerus

These are extra-articular fractures and are produced in one of two ways: flexion or extension. The flexion type is rare after the age of 20.

MECHANISM

Flexion: A force directed against the posterior aspect of the flexed elbow. Extension: A fall on the outstretched arm with hyperextension of the elbow.

CLINICAL PRESENTATION

Pain is severe with marked deformity and swelling. There may appear to be a dislocation, but the triangular relationship of the olecranon and epicondyles is usually maintained. The risk of neurovascular compromise is high.

ROENTGENOGRAMS

AP and lateral (Fig. 5-5) views are sufficient. If the fracture is undisplaced, an anterior fat pad sign will usually be present. Bowman's angle (Fig. 5-6) is altered in this fracture, and comparison to the opposite elbow is helpful. The direction of the displacement of the distal fragment correlates with the type of injury. The distal fragment is posteriorly displaced in the extension injury and anteriorly displaced in the flexion injury. The fracture appears to be transverse on the AP view, but oblique on the lateral view.

COMPLICATIONS

Vascular: This injury may cause arterial compromise and result in ischemic contractures of the forearm. It should be remembered that a compartment syndrome *can develop even in the presence of distal pulses.* Neurologic: The median and ulnar nerves are subject to injury by the fracture fragments. Malunion with loss of the carrying angle can also occur.

TREATMENT

These fractures should be reduced as soon as possible. Skeletal traction with an olecranon pin may be required. Admission to the hospital is advisable after closed reduction to observed the neurovascular system.

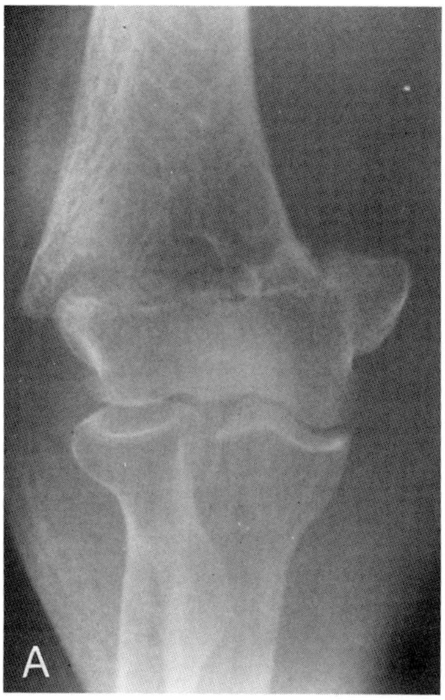

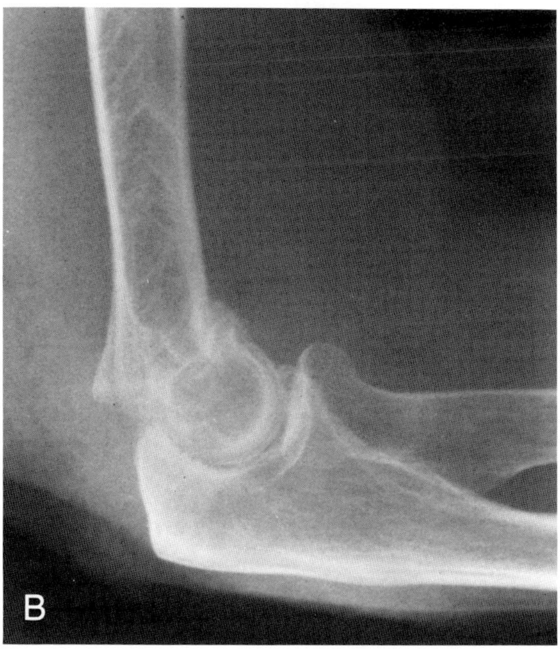

Fig. 5-5. Supracondylar fracture. (A) AP view. (B) Lateral view.

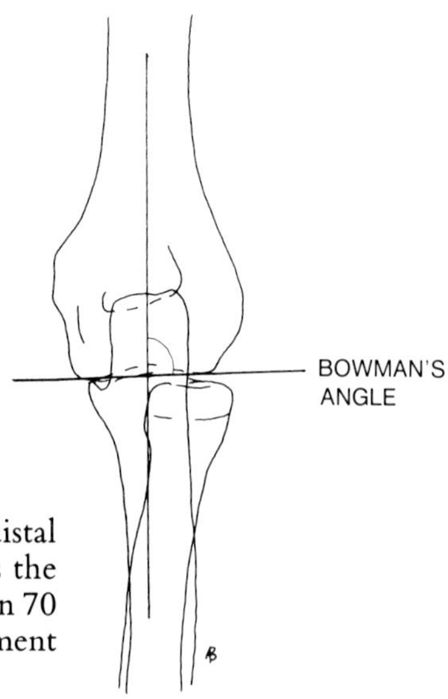

Fig. 5-6. Bowman's angle. The orientation of the distal humeral shaft in relationship to a line drawn across the trochlea and capitellum should form an angle between 70 and 90 degrees. This is helpful in evaluating the alignment and orientation of elbow fractures.

Olecranon Fractures

MECHANISM

A direct blow or a fall on the olecranon may produce a comminuted fracture. Indirect violence, such as a forceful triceps contraction or a fall on the hand with the elbow flexed, will produce a transverse or oblique fracture with lesser degrees of comminution.

CLINICAL PRESENTATION

Effusion, pain, and tenderness are evident. The motion is markedly decreased and the patient may be unable to extend the elbow. A defect in the olecranon can be palpable. In undisplaced fractures, with the triceps aponeurosis intact, the ability to extend the elbow may be maintained.

ROENTGENOGRAMS

AP and lateral views are sufficient, but the lateral view (Fig. 5-7) provides the most information. Fractures with less than 2 mm of displacement can be considered undisplaced. They do not change with flexion, and the patient is usually able to extend the forearm against gravity.

COMPLICATIONS

Radial head fracture or dislocation can occur.

TREATMENT

Undisplaced fractures may be treated with simple immobilization. Displaced fractures require open reduction and internal fixation.

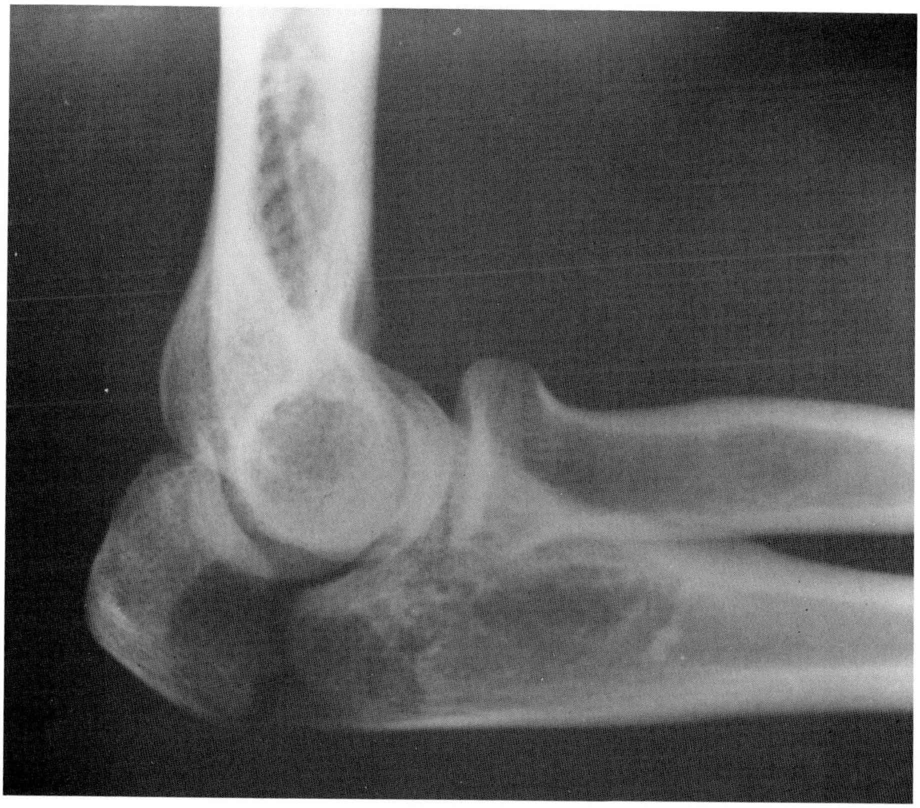

Fig. 5-7. Olecranon process fracture. This is best seen on the lateral view and is often displaced due to the pull of the triceps muscle.

Radial Head Fractures

A fracture of the head or neck of the radius, which is intraarticular, is common in adults.

MECHANISM

This injury results from a fall on the outstretched hand.

CLINICAL PRESENTATION

There is decreased motion, variable degree of swelling, and pain with supination. Tenderness is present over the radial head.

ROENTGENOGRAMS

AP, lateral, and oblique views (Fig. 5-8) are needed, but the fracture often cannot be detected initially. A positive fat pad sign may be present. In any patient with a history of a fall, a positive fat pad sign and a negative roentgenogram, a presumptive diagnosis of an isolated radial head fracture should be made. Repeat roentgenograms in 7 to 10 days are recommended.

COMPLICATIONS

Associated hand, wrist or capitellar fractures may be present.

TREATMENT

The arm should be immobilized in a posterior splint. If severly comminuted or displaced, the radial head may need to be excised.

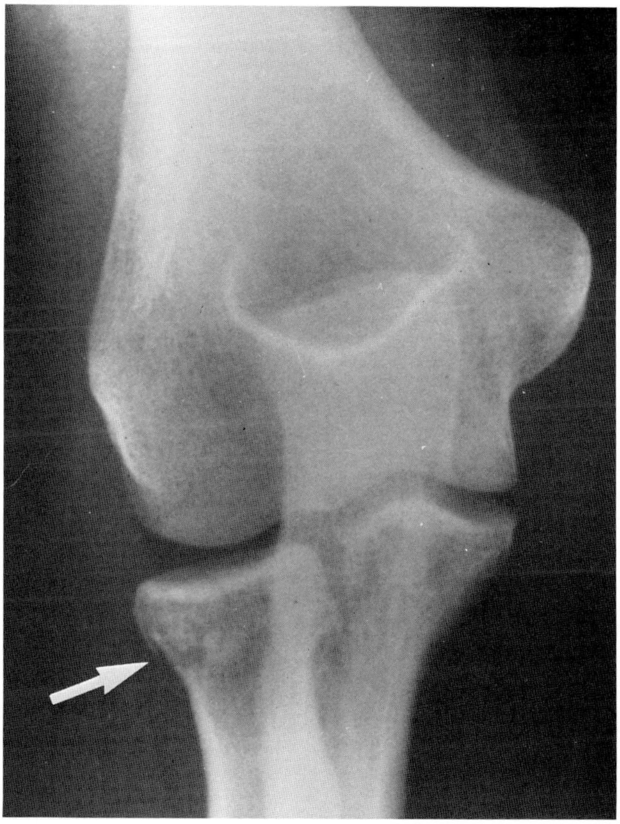

Fig. 5-8. Radial neck fracture. This may be seen well on the AP or the oblique view (arrow).

Elbow Dislocations

This is the third most commonly dislocated joint, after the shoulder and the fingers. The most common type of elbow dislocation (80 to 90%) is the posterior or posterolateral dislocation.

MECHANISM

The dislocation is produced by a fall on the outstretched arm with the elbow and the arm abducted.

CLINICAL PRESENTATION

There is often massive swelling due to the extensive soft tissue injury. The elbow is held in 45 degrees of flexion. The triangular relationship of the olecranon and the epicondyles is lost. The olecranon is prominent posteriorly.

ROENTGENOGRAMS

AP, lateral, and oblique views are needed (Fig. 5-9) to rule out any associated fractures and to assess the joint thoroughly. The radius and ulna lie posterior and lateral to the humerus, and the radius is not aligned with the capitellum.

TREATMENT

The elbow should be reduced as soon as possible with longitudinal traction and pressure over the olecranon. The elbow should be kept in flexion after reduction to maintain the reduction. Open reduction is rarely necessary, but repeated attempts at a closed reduction increase the damage to the soft tissues.

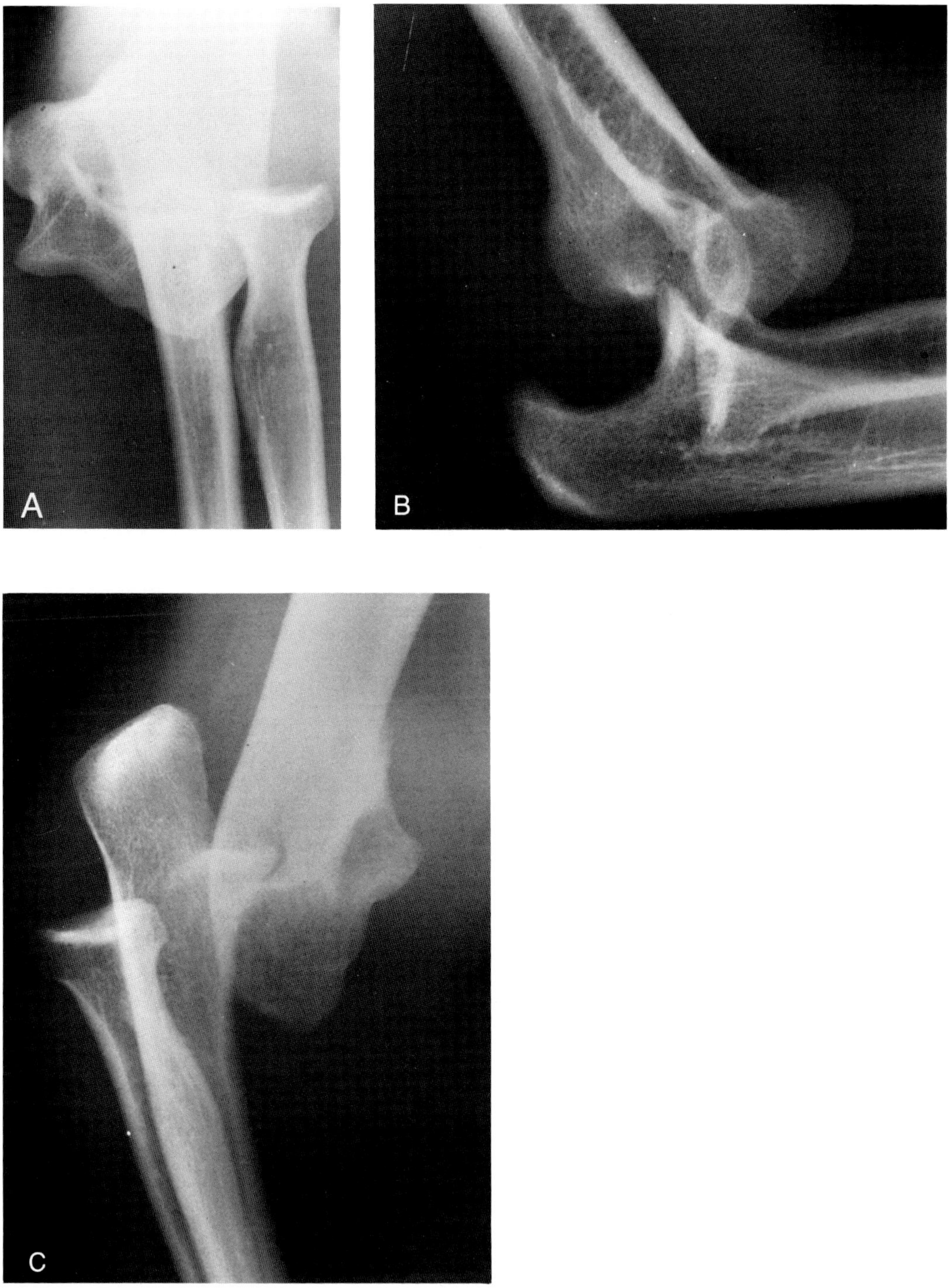

Fig. 5-9. Elbow dislocation. (A) AP view. (B) Lateral view. (C) Oblique view. There is disruption in the normal anatomical alignment.

Anterior Dislocation

This is extremely rare.

MECHANISM

A direct blow to the olecranon, driving it anteriorly, produces this dislocation.

CLINICAL PRESENTATION

The elbow is extended with the arm shortened and the forearm elongated. The biceps tendon is prominent anteriorly and a void is felt in the olecranon fossa.

ROENTGENOGRAMS

AP, lateral, and oblique films show the olecranon resting on the anterior surface of the humerus. The relationship of the radius to the capitellum and the olecranon to the epicondyles is lost.

TREATMENT

Reduction should be performed as soon as possible.

Radial Head Dislocation

This dislocation is rare in adults.

MECHANISM

A fall on the pronated forearm with the elbow flexed levers the radius anteriorly. A blow to the anterior forearm may dislocate the radius posterially.

CLINICAL PRESENTATION

There is pain and swelling with the forearm held in pronation.

ROENTGENOGRAMS

AP, lateral, and oblique views (Fig. 5-10) are taken, including the entire ulna so that an associated ulnar fracture is not missed. The radial-capitellar alignment is lost.

COMPLICATIONS

Associated fractures commonly include an avulsion of the epicondyle or coronoid process. The avulsed fragments can be displaced into the joint. Neuropraxia of the ulnar nerve can occur. Brachial artery injury occurs in 4 percent of cases. If the pulse disappears after reduction, decreasing the elbow flexion will usually relieve the pressure on the artery. If not, an immediate arteriogram is indicated.

TREATMENT

Reduction as soon as possible followed by placing the arm in a strong posterior splint. A circumferential cast should not be used, since significant swelling may occur.

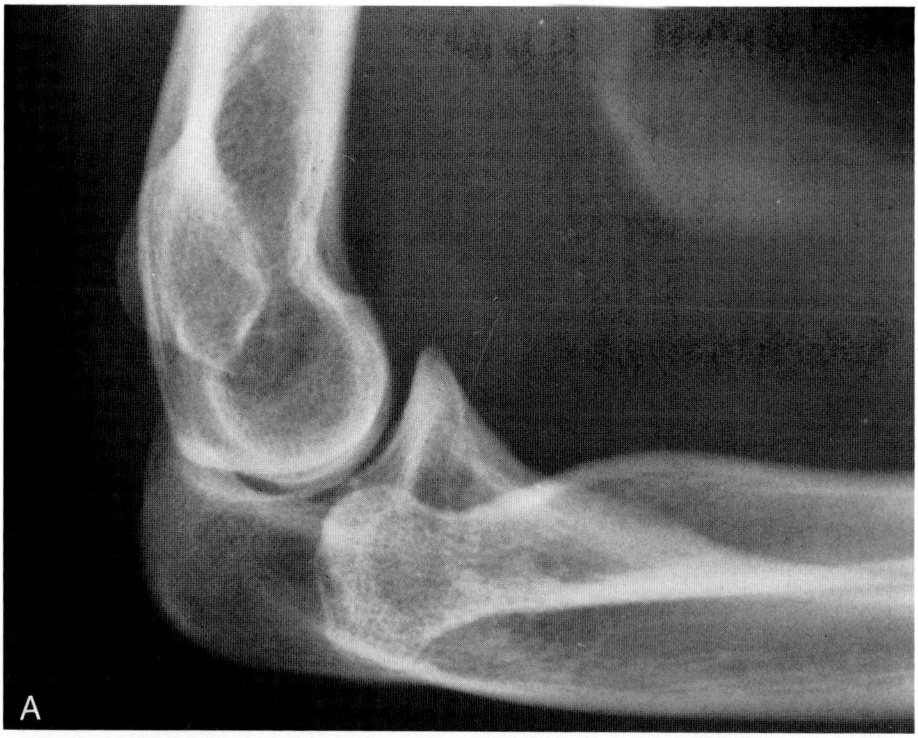

Fig. 5-10. (A) Posterior dislocation of the radius. (A) AP view (Figure continues).

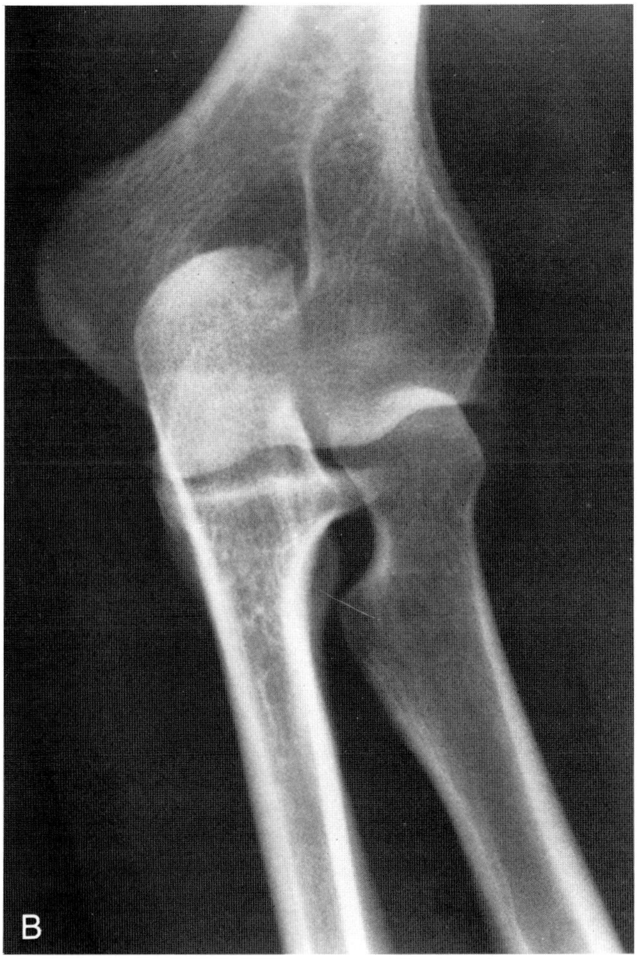

Fig. 5-10 (Continued). (B) Oblique view. Note that a line drawn down the shaft of the radius does not intersect the capitellum.

6
The Forearm

Fractures of the radius and ulna between the elbow and the wrist arise from a wide range of deforming forces. Routine radiographs include an AP (Fig. 6-1A) and a lateral (Fig. 6-1B) view. Both the elbow and the wrist should always be visualized on the radiographs.

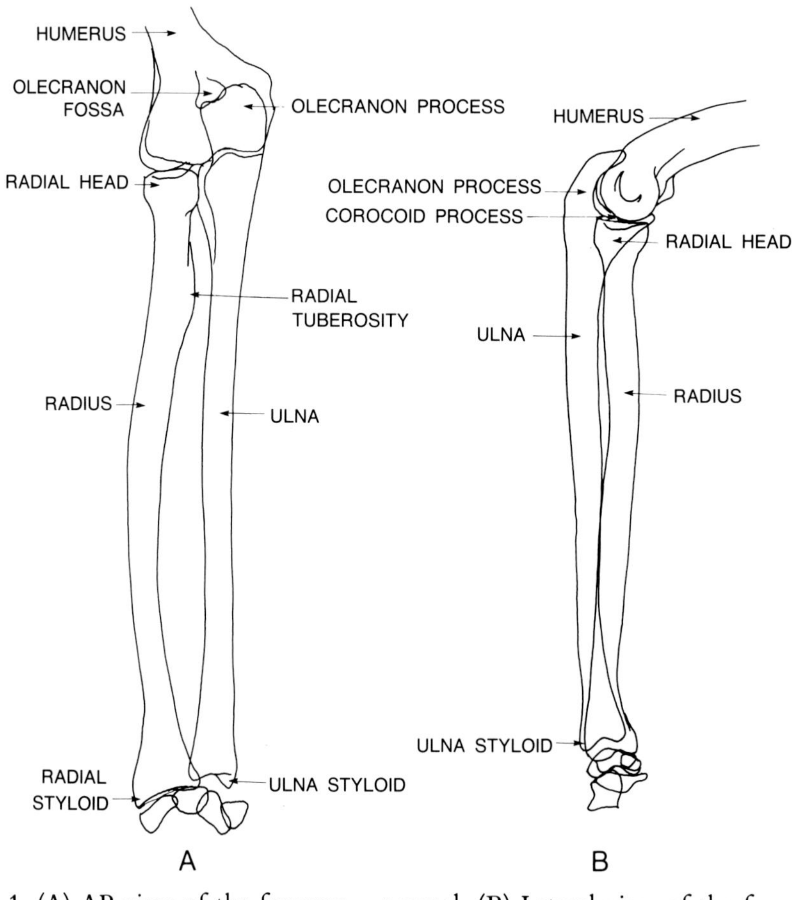

Fig. 6-1. (A) AP view of the forearm — normal. (B) Lateral view of the forearm — normal (Figure continues).

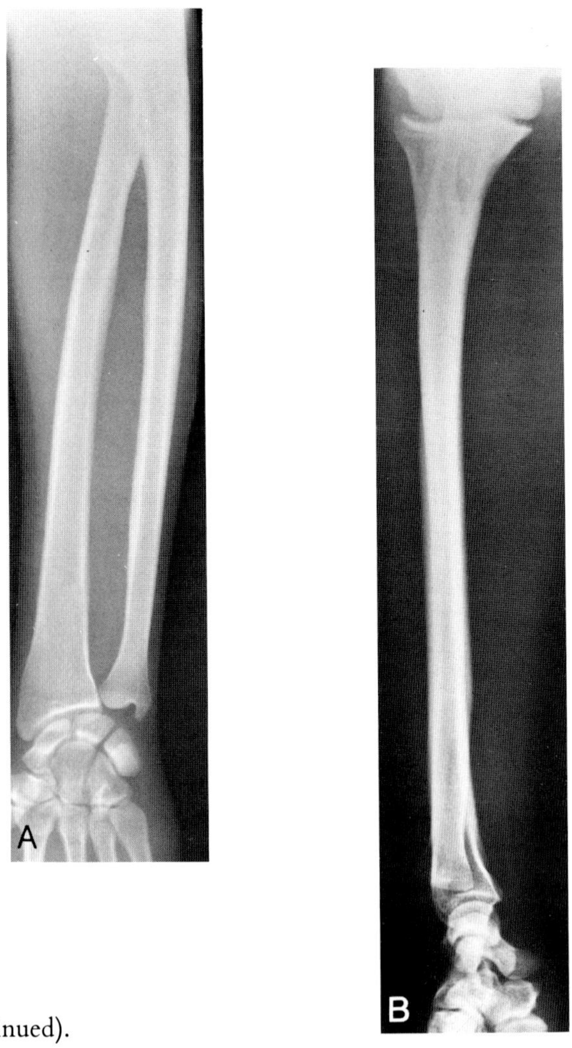

Fig. 6-1 (Continued).

Monteggia Fractures

This is a fracture of the proximal third of the ulna, associated with dislocation of the radial head. It constitutes 7 percent of the radial and ulnar fractures.

MECHANISM

A fall on the outstretched arm with rotation, usually pronation, causes the ulna to fracture and levers the radius anteriorly.

CLINICAL PRESENTATION

There is pain and inability to move the elbow. Gross swelling and deformity of the elbow and proximal forearm are present.

ROENTGENOGRAMS

AP, lateral, and oblique views (Fig. 6-2) show the fracture of the ulna and the radial head dislocation. The radial head-capitellar alignment is lost. This part of the injury is often missed.

COMPLICATIONS

Twenty percent of patients with this fracture have radial nerve palsy. Associated injuries to the wrist can occur.

TREATMENT

Reduction of the radial head dislocation with gentle supination as soon as possible. The ulnar fracture usually needs open reduction, internal fixation in adults. Reduction of the radial head may be difficult to maintain without reduction of the proximal ulnar fracture.

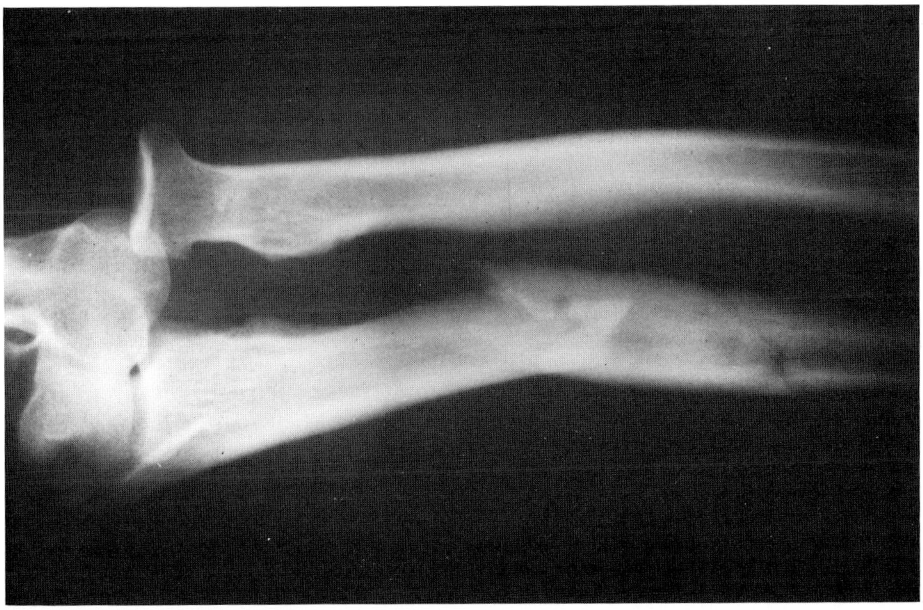

Fig. 6-2. Monteggia fracture dislocation of the elbow. There is a dislocation of the radius at the elbow joint and a fracture of the proximal third of the ulna.

RADIUS

Fracture of the proximal two-thirds of the radius in adults is rare without an associated ulnar fracture. An isolated fracture at the junction of the middle and distal thirds can occur.

Fracture of Radius and Ulna (Both-Bones Fracture)

The deformity of the fracture is determined by the location of the fracture and the resultant muscular pull.

MECHANISM

A violent blow to the forearm is a common etiology. Athletic injuries with a fall can also produce the fracture.

CLINICAL PRESENTATION

Pain, swelling and obvious deformity of the forearm are present.

ROENTGENOGRAMS

AP and lateral views (Fig. 6-3) are useful to determine comminution, angulation, shortening, and rotation. As with all forearm injuries, the wrist and elbow must be examined—but not necessarily on the same radiograph.

COMPLICATIONS

A compartment syndrome can develop in the forearm, either after injury, reduction, or surgery. Increasing pain with passive extension of the fingers and the thumb is the most reliable sign of an impending compartment syndrome. It should again be emphasized that pulses may be normal even in the presence of a compartment syndrome. Release of the dressings should be done immediately, and a fasciotomy may prove to be necessary.

TREATMENT

Closed reduction may be successful, but often leads to malunion or delayed union in adults. Open reduction and internal fixation is the preferred treatment, except in children.

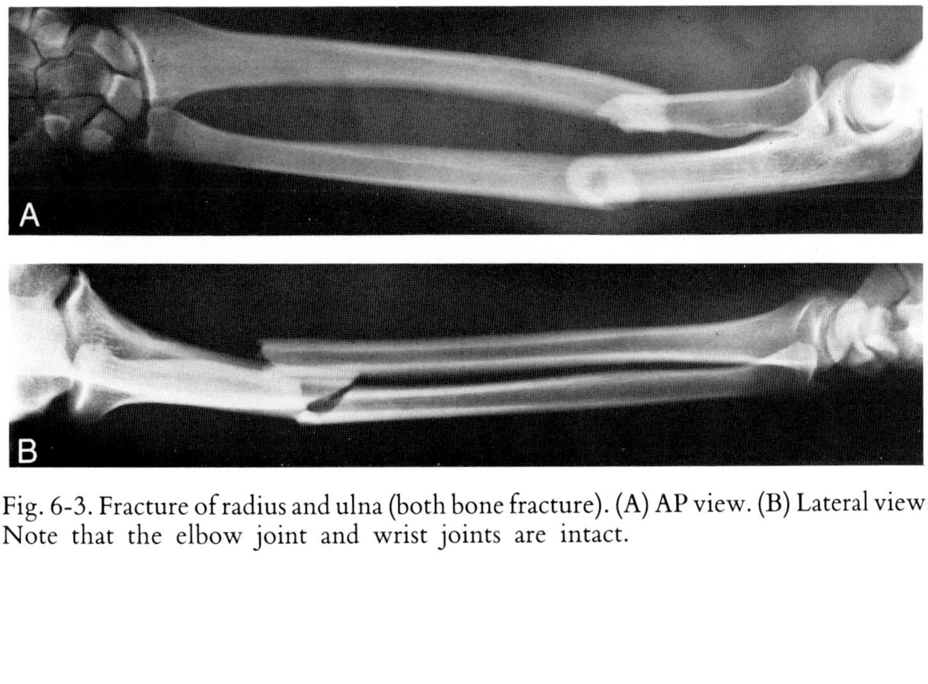

Fig. 6-3. Fracture of radius and ulna (both bone fracture). (A) AP view. (B) Lateral view. Note that the elbow joint and wrist joints are intact.

Ulnar Fracture (Nightstick Fracture)

This fracture is a nondisplaced or slightly displaced fracture of the shaft of the ulna.

MECHANISM

As the name suggests, the etiology is usually a direct blow.

CLINICAL PRESENTATION

There is pain and localized tenderness over the ulna. The history should reveal direct violence to the forearm.

ROENTGENOGRAMS

AP and lateral views (Fig. 6-4) are usually satisfactory. If the fragments are displaced, a fracture of the radius or a dislocation at the wrist or elbow should be suspected.

COMPLICATIONS

These are rare.

TREATMENT

A cast for immobilization is necessary.

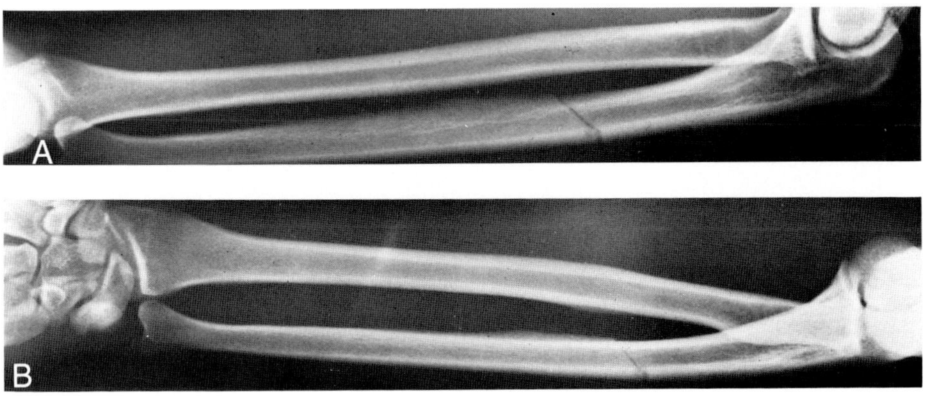

Fig. 6-4. Nightstick fracture. (A) Lateral view. (B) AP view. The fracture is nondisplaced and the radial head is located.

Fracture of the Middle and Distal Thirds

MECHANISM

A fall on the outstretched hand with a rotational force is usually responsible for these fractures.

CLINICAL PRESENTATION

Pain and swelling of the distal forearm are present. Wrist and hand motion are quite painful, and function of the distal radio-ulnar joint is reduced.

ROENTGENOGRAMS

AP, lateral, and oblique views must demonstrate the distal radio-ulnar joint to be reduced. The radius may be slightly dorsally displaced and shortened.

COMPLICATIONS

Missing dislocation of the distal radio-ulnar joint is the most likely complication.

TREATMENT

This fracture should be treated by closed reduction in a long-arm cast with the forearm in pronation. Open reduction may be necessary.

Galleazzi Fracture Dislocation

This injury is a fracture of the distal radius with a dislocation of the distal radio-ulnar joints. The ulnar styloid may or may not be fractured. It is three times more common than the Monteggia fracture, but often misdiagnosed.

MECHANISM

A direct blow to the dorsolateral side of the wrist, or fall on the outstretched arm with pronation of the forearm, produces this injury.

CLINICAL PRESENTATION

The forearm is shortened with a concave deformity on the radial side. The wrist is swollen and painful and the ulnar head may be prominent.

ROENTGENOGRAMS

AP and lateral views (Fig. 6-5) of the entire forearm are needed, including the elbow and wrist joints. The radial fracture usually occurs at the junction of the

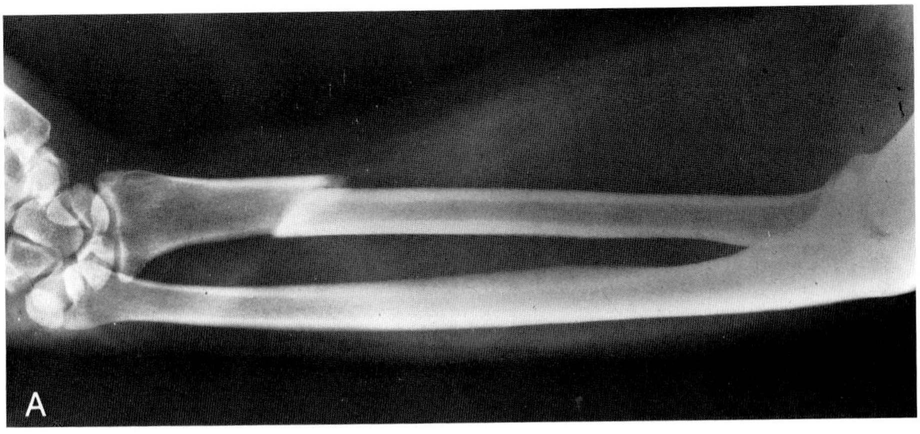

Fig. 6-5. Galeazzi fracture dislocation. (A) The AP view appears minimally displaced (Figure continues).

middle and distal thirds of the radius. An ulnar styloid fracture may or may not be present. The space at the distal radial ulnar joint is widened. The ulna can be displaced dorsally or volarly.

COMPLICATIONS

Loss of reduction with closed treatment.

TREATMENT

Open reduction and internal fixation is usually required in adults, since this injury has been known to displace, even in a long-arm cast.

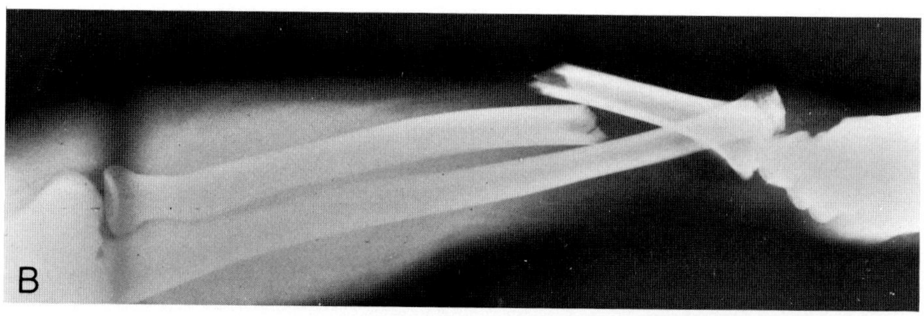

Fig. 6-5 (Continued). (B) The lateral view depicts significant displacement of the fracture as well as the obvious dislocation of the distal radial-ulnar joint.

7 The Wrist

The wrist encompasses the distal radius and ulna as well as the eight carpal bones. Since most of this area is covered with articular cartilage, fractures of these bones are usually intra-articular with the potential for wrist disorders in the future. Sixty percent of the distal radius fractures are the "Colles' variety" and 50 percent of the carpal fractures involve the scaphoid bone. Carpal fractures account for 6 percent of all fractures. AP (Fig. 7-1A), lateral (Fig. 7-1B) and oblique (Fig. 7-1C) views are the minimum radiographs necessary to evaluate a wrist injury. A carpal tunnel view (Fig. 7-1D) may also be of help.

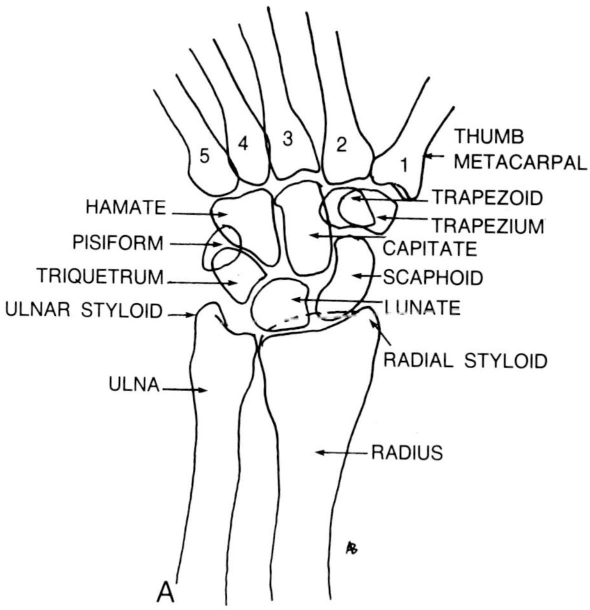

A

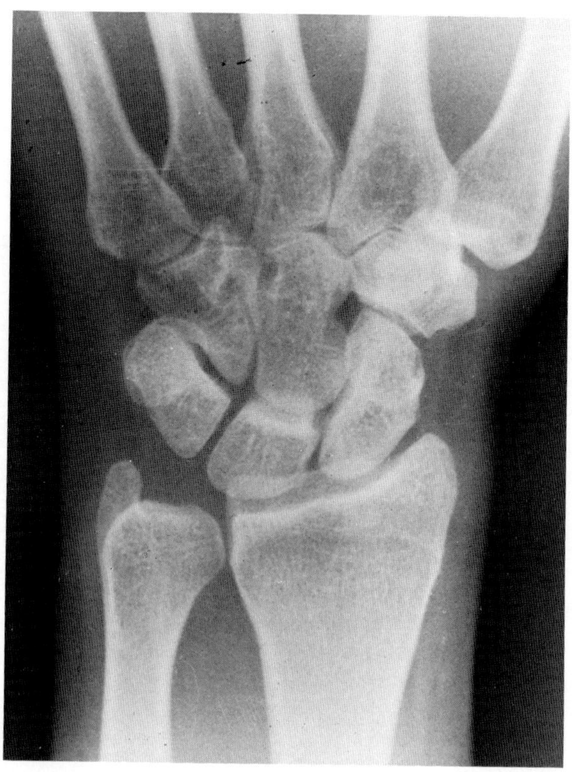

A

Fig. 7-1. (A) AP view of the wrist — normal (Continues).

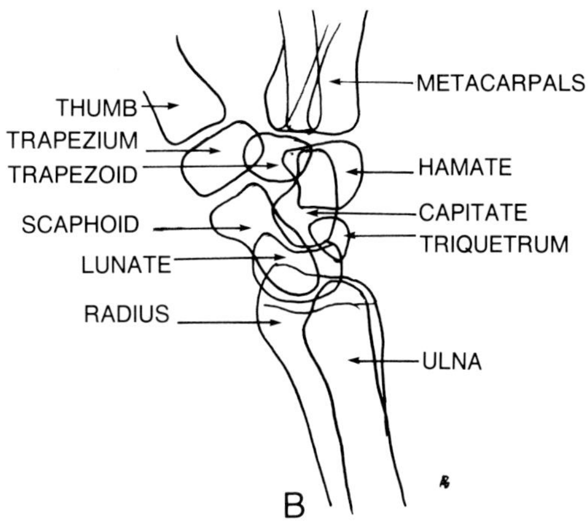

B

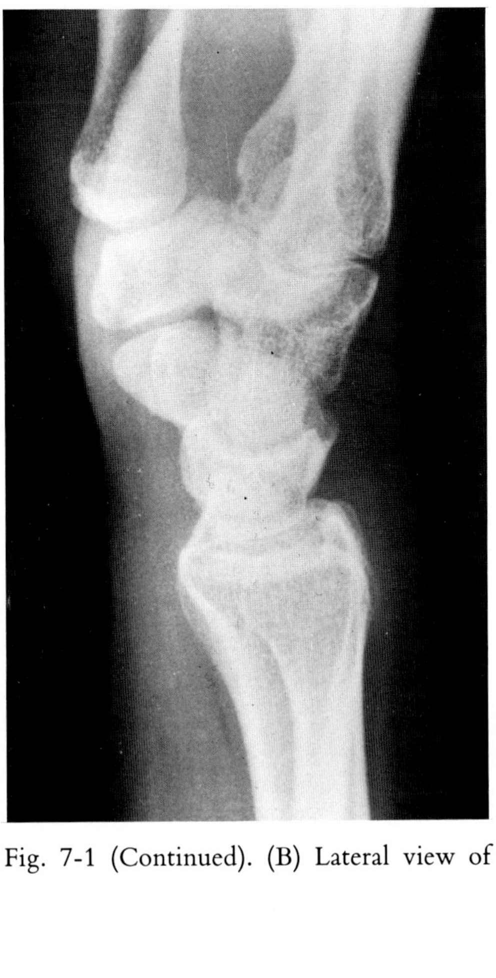

Fig. 7-1 (Continued). (B) Lateral view of the wrist—normal (Continues).

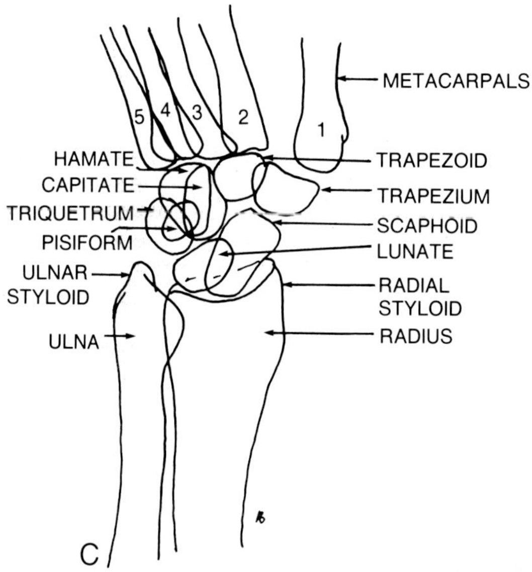

C

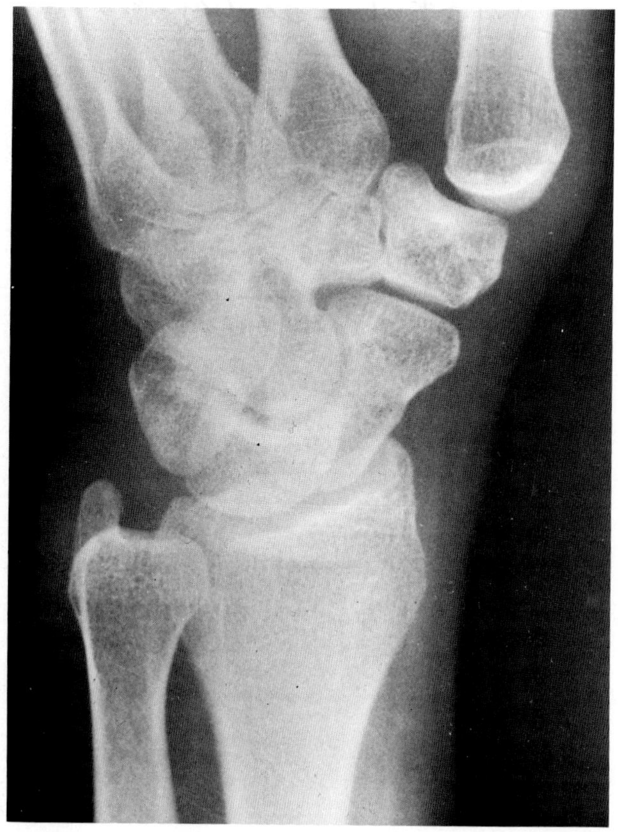

Fig. 7-1 (C) (Continued). C

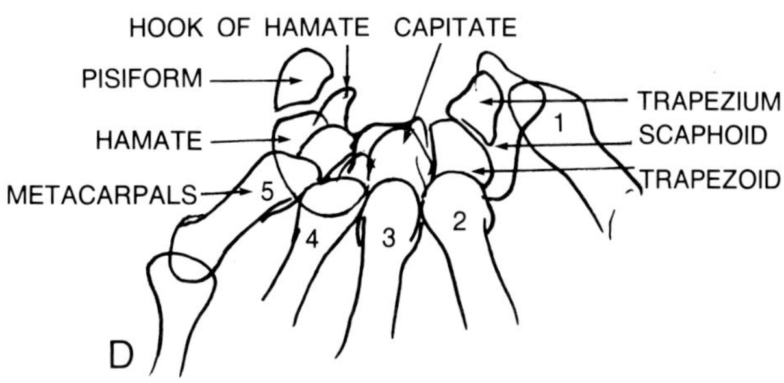

D

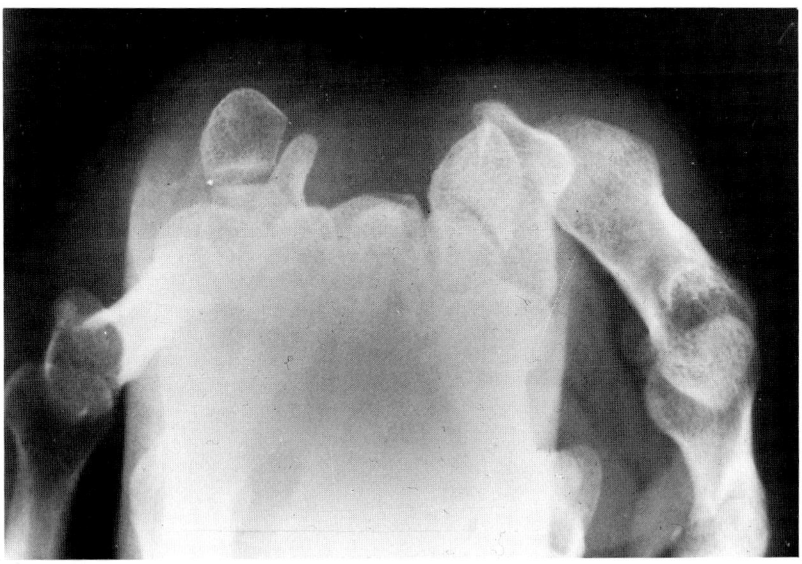

D

Fig. 7-1 (Continued). (C) Oblique view of the wrist — normal. (D) Carpal tunnel view of the wrist — normal.

Wrist Check List (Normal Anatomic Relationship)

10 degrees of volar tilt of the distal radius (Fig. 7-2).
20 degrees of radial deviation (Fig. 7-3A).
12 mm from the radial styloid to the articular edge of the radius (Fig. 7-3A).
0 degrees capitolunate angle. A straight line down the third metacarpal, capitate, lunate, and shaft of the radius when the wrist is in neutral position (Fig. 7-4).
47 degrees scapholunate angle. 30 to 70 degrees normal variation range (Fig. 7-5A).
Less than 2 mm space at the scapholunate joint (Fig. 7-5B).

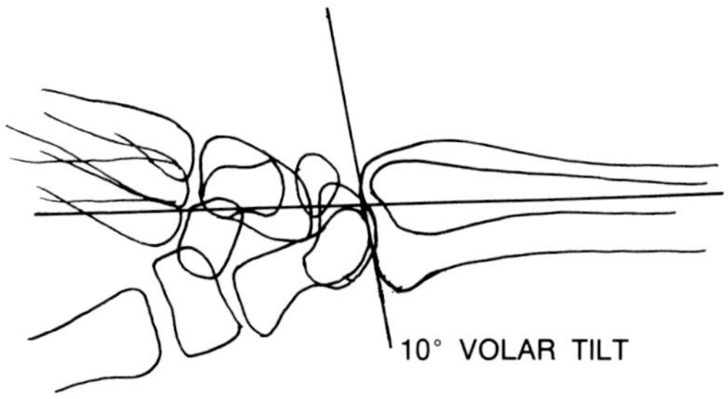

Fig. 7-2. The articular end of the radius has a volar inclination of 10 degrees to a line drawn down the shaft of the radius.

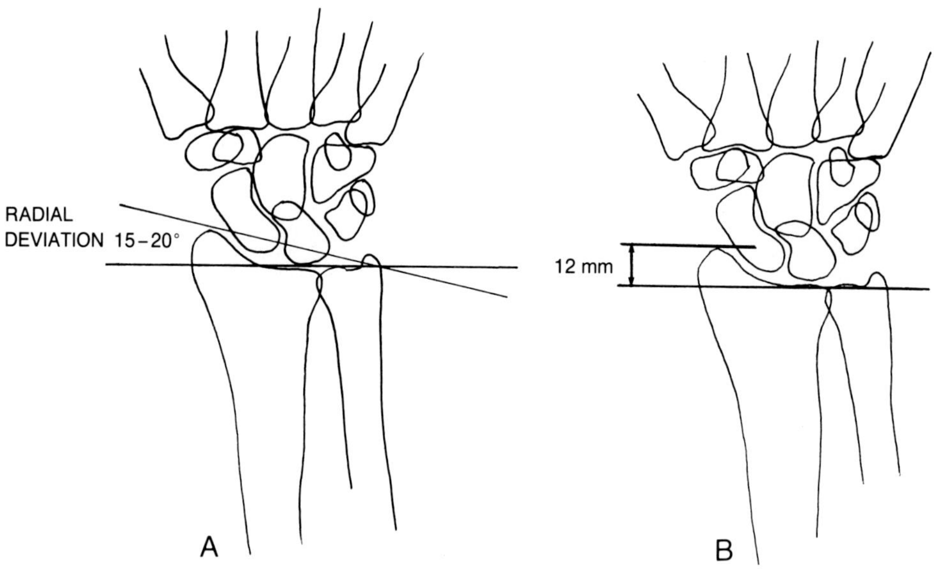

Fig. 7-3. (A) An angle of 20 degrees is formed between the distal end of the radius and a line drawn down the shaft of the radius. (B) The radial styloid should be 12 mm from the articular edge of the radius.

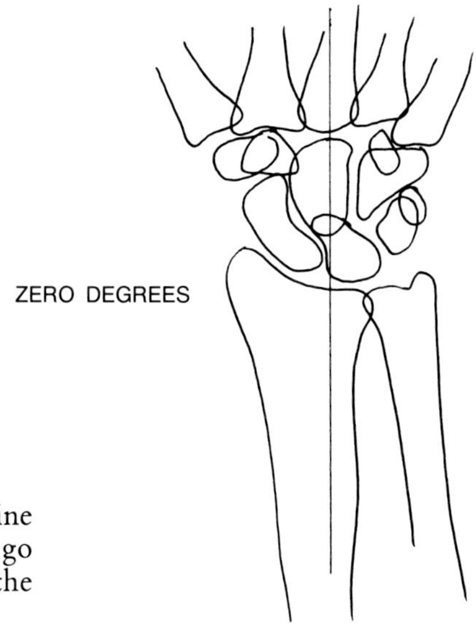

Fig. 7-4. Capitolunate angle. A straight line down the third metacarpal should go through lunate, capitate, and the shaft of the radius, in a straight line.

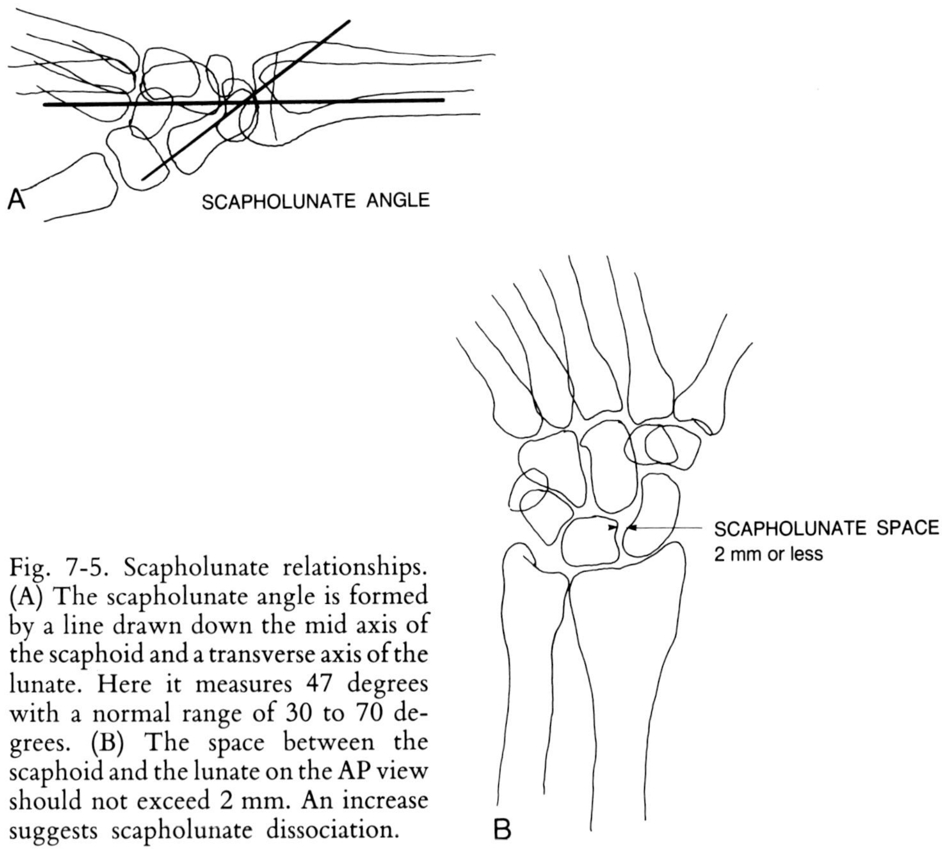

Fig. 7-5. Scapholunate relationships. (A) The scapholunate angle is formed by a line drawn down the mid axis of the scaphoid and a transverse axis of the lunate. Here it measures 47 degrees with a normal range of 30 to 70 degrees. (B) The space between the scaphoid and the lunate on the AP view should not exceed 2 mm. An increase suggests scapholunate dissociation.

Colles' Fracture

This is the most common wrist injury. It accounts for 60 percent of distal radius fractures.

MECHANISM

A fall on the outstretched arm with the hand in dorsiflexion and pronation of the forearm about the fixed hand. Impaction of the lunate on the radius causes the intra-articular fracture of the radius.

CLINICAL PRESENTATION

The characteristic configuration is the "silver fork" deformity of the wrist from the dorsal displacement of the fracture. There is significant pain, tenderness, swelling, and weakness. There may be altered sensibility in either the median or ulnar nerve distribution.

ROENTGENOGRAMS

AP and lateral views (Fig. 7-6) are the bare minimum needed, but the addition of an oblique film is helpful. There is an ulnar styloid fracture in 60 percent of cases. Associated fracture of the carpal bones can occur. Associated elbow fractures are less common but the elbow should be evaluated if there is the slightest suspicion of injury. The radial fracture is seen to be: (1) dorsally and laterally displaced (radial deviation), (2) shortened or impacted, (3) supinated, and (4) occasionally intra-articular (radio-ulnar or radiocarpal).

COMPLICATIONS

A carpal tunnel syndrome can result from contusion of the median nerve or hemorrhage into the carpal canal. Ulnar nerve injury is less common. Inadequate reduction is a frequent occurrence.

TREATMENT

Reduction and immobilization in a long-arm splint or cast is necessary. Open reduction or pins-in-plaster or external fixation may be necessary, if an acceptable reduction cannot be achieved and maintained.

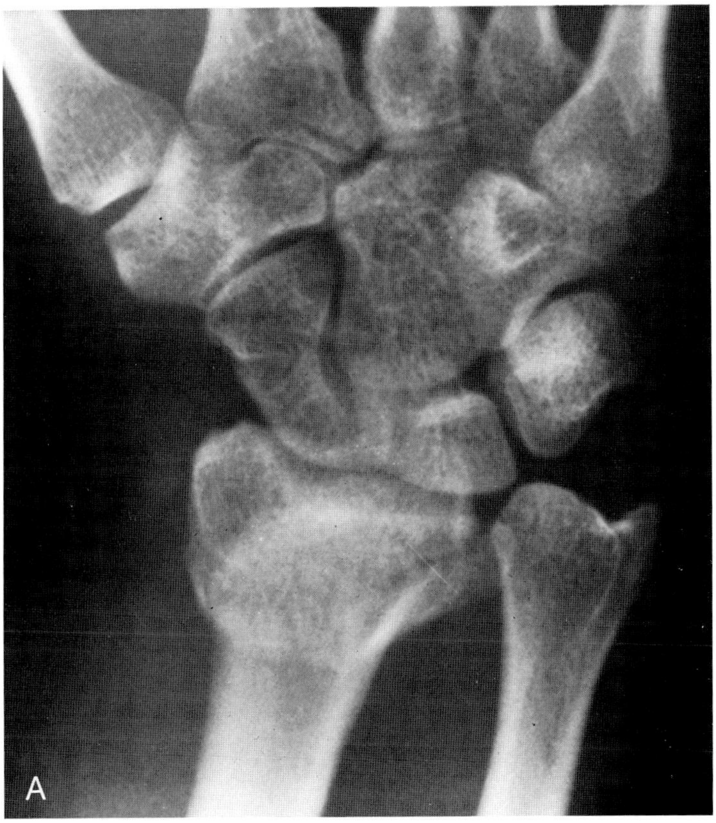

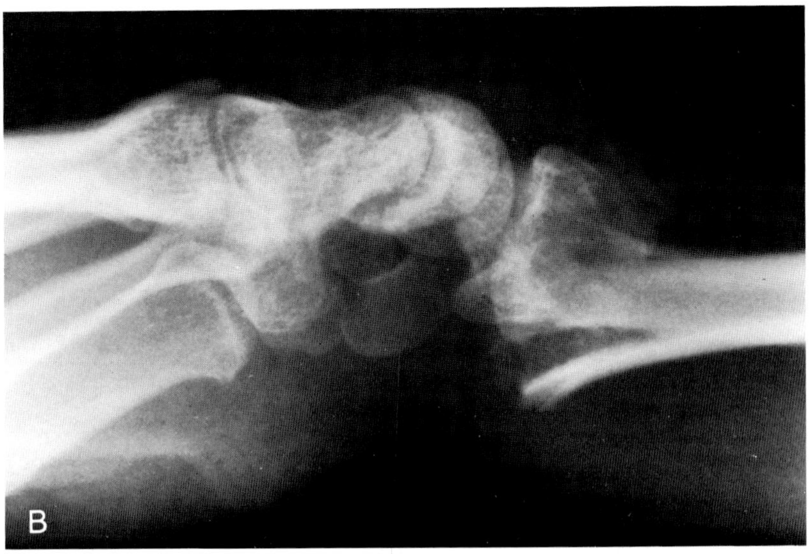

Fig. 7-6. Colles' fracture. (A) AP view. (B) Lateral view reveals the classical dorsal displacement and angulation.

Smith's Fracture

This is an injury with volar displacement of distal fragments. It is much less common than a Colles' fracture.

MECHANISM

A fall on the dorsiflexed hand with supination of the forearm on the fixed wrist produces the fracture.

CLINICAL PRESENTATION

The patient presents with a reverse "silver fork" deformity. There is significant pain, swelling, and tenderness.

ROENTGENOGRAMS

AP, lateral, and oblique views (Fig. 7-7) should be obtained. The distal radius is displaced volarly. The injury is often intra-articular. Ulnar styloid fractures frequently accompany this fracture. Other carpal fractures may also coexist but are less common.

COMPLICATIONS

Misdiagnosis as a Colles' fracture occurs, as well as improper reduction and immobilization.

TREATMENT

Closed reduction in a long-arm cast with the hand supinated is necessary.

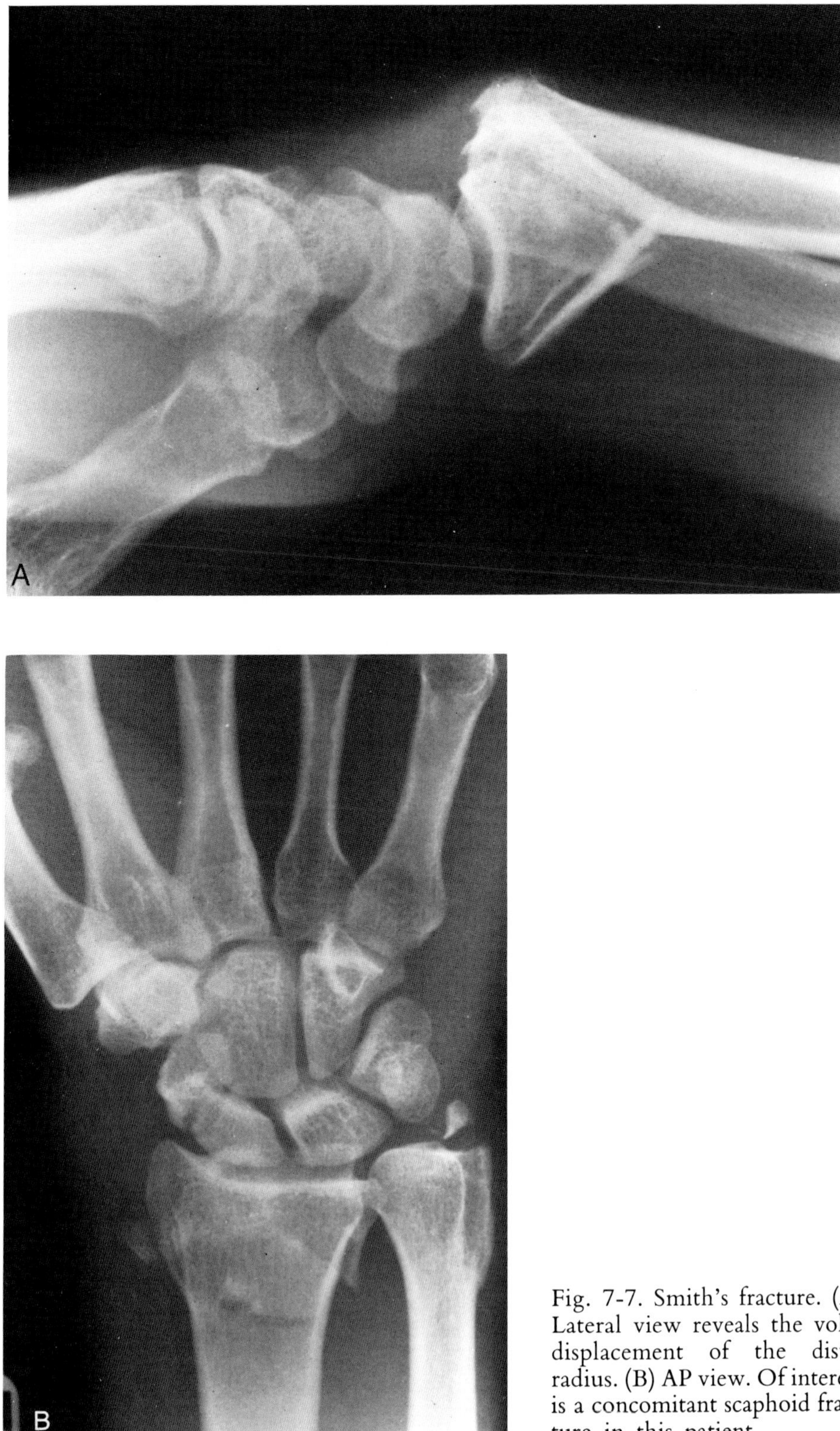

Fig. 7-7. Smith's fracture. (A) Lateral view reveals the volar displacement of the distal radius. (B) AP view. Of interest is a concomitant scaphoid fracture in this patient.

Barton's Fracture

A Barton's fracture is an intra-articular fracture of either the dorsal or volar articular surface of the distal radius.

MECHANISM

A fall on the outstretched arm with the hand in dorsiflexion produces a volar surface injury, while a fall with flexion of the wrist produces the dorsal surface fractures.

CLINICAL PRESENTATION

Pain, swelling, and deformity of the wrist are present.

ROENTGENOGRAMS

The lateral view (Fig. 7-8) provides the most information, but obviously an AP view is necessary to exclude other fractures. The carpus is displaced dorsally or volarly, depending on the direction of the injury, with the lunate settling into the fracture defect.

COMPLICATIONS

Median nerve damage is less common than with a Colles' fracture.

TREATMENT

Closed reduction should be attempted, but open reduction and internal fixation is indicated if closed reduction is unsuccessful.

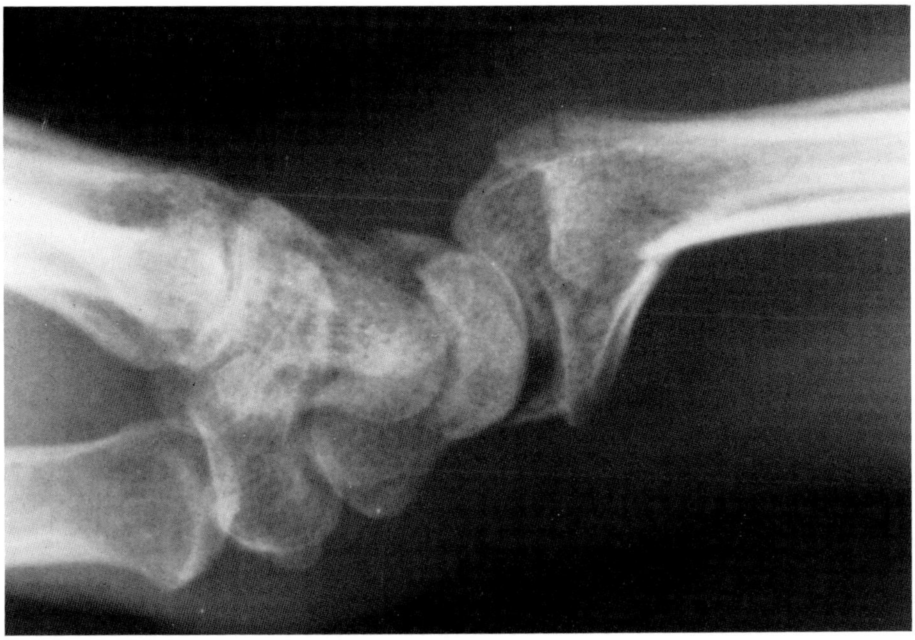

Fig. 7-8. Volar Barton's fracture. This is a fracture through the articular surface in the volar plane of the distal radius. There is volar subluxation of the carpus.

Scaphoid Fractures

Scaphoid fractures account for 60 to 70 percent of carpal fractures. The diagnosis is based on clinical as well as roentgenographic findings. Because of the vascular supply, a high incidence of avascular necrosis or non-union exists. When treated appropriately, 90 percent of scaphoid fractures will heal. If the initial roentgenograms are normal, the wrist should be splinted and repeat roentgenograms performed in 10 to 14 days.

MECHANISM

A fall on the outstretched hand is the most common mechanism of injury.

CLINICAL PRESENTATION

Swelling of the wrist and pain in the anatomical snuff box, just distal to Lister's tubercle, should lead to a suspicion of a scaphoid fracture.

ROENTGENOGRAMS

AP, lateral, oblique, and scaphoid views (Fig. 7-9) will demonstrate the majority of visible fractures. Unfortunately, not all acute scaphoid fractures are roentgenographically apparent initially. This is another reason to treat a clinically suspected scaphoid fracture with a negative roentgenogram. Repeat roentgeno-

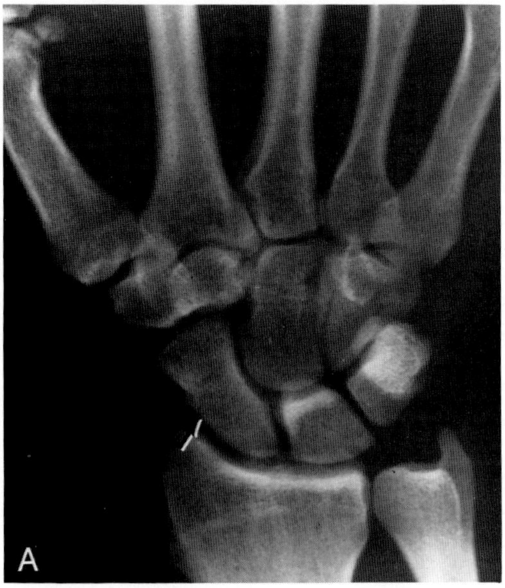

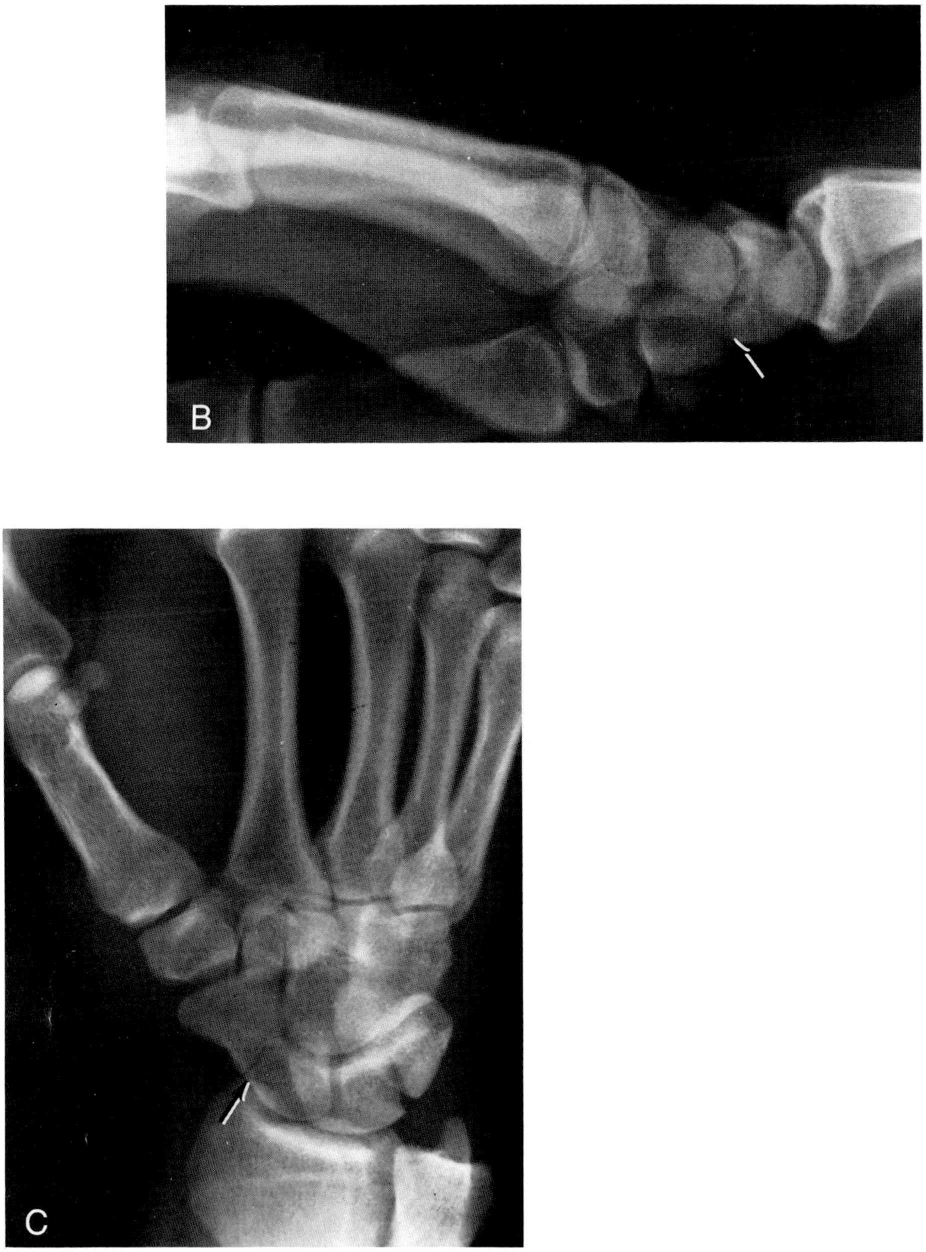

Fig. 7-9. Scaphoid fracture (arrow).

grams in two weeks will often show the fracture. The majority of scaphoid fractures occur at its waist.

COMPLICATIONS

Misdiagnosis is the most frequent problem, which increases the incidence of non-union and avascular necrosis. The risk of avascular necrosis increases with the more proximal location of the fracture. Concomitant fractures of the hand, distal radius, or radial head should not be overlooked, and roentgenograms of these areas should be obtained if clinically indicated.

TREATMENT

Fractures or suspected fractures should be placed in a thumb spica cast. Controversy exists over long-arm or short-arm immobilization. Repeat roentgenograms should be done on suspected fractures in 10 to 14 days.

Lunate Fractures

Lunate fractures account for approximately 3 percent of carpal fractures.

MECHANISM

A fall on the heel of the hand with the wrist dorsiflexed produces an osteochondral shear fracture.

CLINICAL PRESENTATION

There is pain and weakness of wrist function with decreased motion. Tenderness over the lunate can be elicited.

ROENTGENOGRAMS

AP and oblique views are the best to see the fracture because there is significant overlap of the carpal bones on the lateral view. The fracture is often difficult to visualize due to superimposition of the radius.

COMPLICATIONS

Osteonecrosis (Kienböck's disease) may develop, especially if the injury is unrecognized. Misdiagnosis of perilunate dislocation or scaphoid fractures should be avoided.

TREATMENT

Immobilization of the wrist with a short-arm cast or splint is useful to provide comfort.

Other Carpal Fractures (Excluding Scaphoid-Lunate)

MECHANISM

Hyperextension of the wrist with a fall on the hand produces most carpal fractures.

CLINICAL PRESENTATION

Pain, swelling and tenderness may be localized to the bone/bones involved.

ROENTGENOGRAMS

AP, lateral, and oblique views are satisfactory for most injuries. The frequency of fractures seen is: a dorsal chip fracture, mainly the triquetrium (Fig. 7-10) followed by fracture of the trapezium. Carpal tunnel view (Fig. 7-11) is best to see fractures of the hook of the hamate.

COMPLICATIONS

Rare.

TREATMENT

Short arm immobilization in a cast or splint is acceptable.

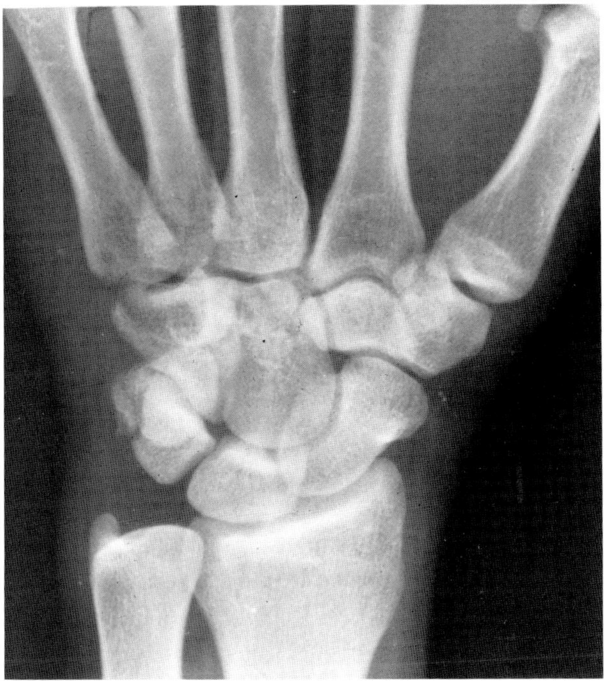

Fig. 7-10. Triquetrium fracture.

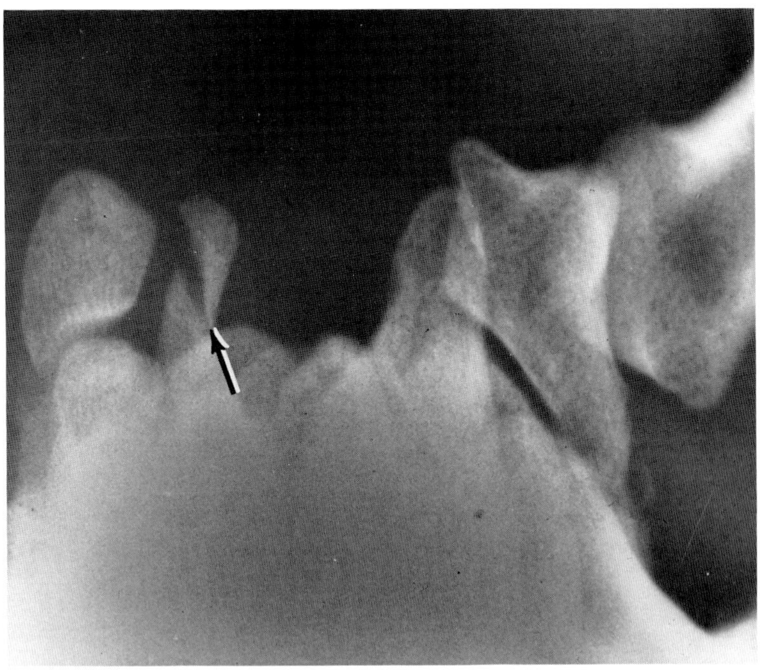

Fig. 7-11. Fracture of the hook of the hamate (arrow) on carpal tunnel view.

Scapholunate Dissociation (Rotary Subluxation of the Scaphoid)

This injury represents one of the most complex of the dorsiflexion wrist instability injuries. It may present as a "sprain" but can carry the sequelae of permanent pain and instability.

MECHANISM

A fall on the dorsiflexed wrist is a common etiology.

CLINICAL PRESENTATION

The patient presents with pain and swelling of his wrist which may or may not be localized to the scaphoid or the scapholunate joint. Swelling may be minimal.

ROENTGENOGRAMS

AP, lateral, and oblique roentgenograms may appear normal. Careful examination of the routine films, the addition of radial and ulnar deviation films, and an AP with the fist clenched will help to demonstrate this complex instability. In examining the radiographs, one should look for (1) an increase in the normal 2 mm space between the scaphoid and the lunate (Fig. 7-12A), (2) a foreshortened appearance of the scaphoid with "cortical ring" shadow on the AP view, which represents abnormal rotation of the scaphoid (Fig. 7-12B), (3) on the lateral view, an abnormal scapholunate angle (Fig. 7-12C) of greater than 70 degrees.

COMPLICATIONS

Wrist instability and pain may be long-term complications of this injury. It is also imperative not to miss an associated carpal or other fracture.

TREATMENT

Early repair of the ligamentous ruptures offers the best chance for a useful wrist.

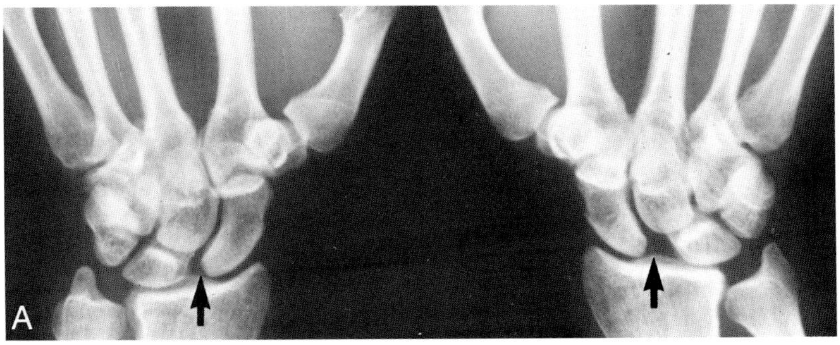

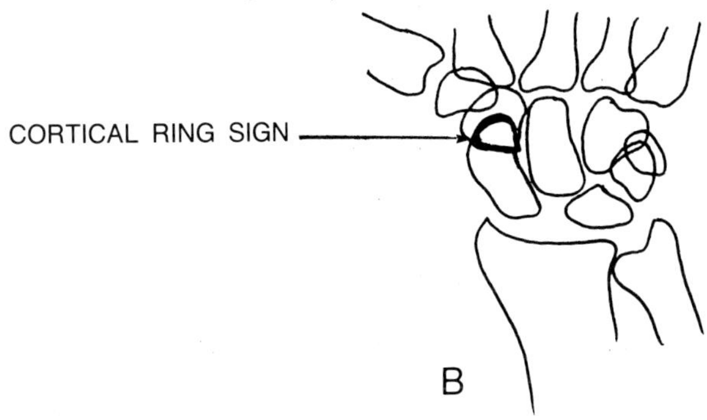

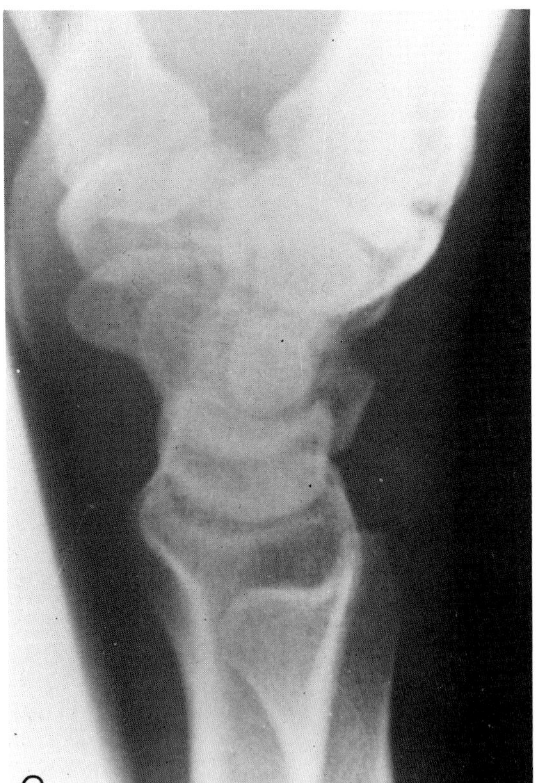

Fig. 7-12. Scapholunate dissociation. (A) The clenched fist AP view reveals the "Terry-Thomas" sign. An increase in the space between the scaphoid and the lunate. (B) The cortical ring sign, due to overlapping of the scaphoid and lesser multangular. (C) An increase in the scapholunate angle is evident on the lateral view.

CARPAL DISLOCATIONS

Each carpal bone has been reported as being dislocated individually. The most common dislocations are lunate or perilunate.

MECHANISM

A fall on the outstretched hand with marked hyperextension of the wrist.

CLINICAL PRESENTATION

The wrist is swollen and tender. Any motion of the wrist is painful. Minimal deformity may be present.

ROENTGENOGRAMS

AP, lateral, and oblique views will reveal the dislocation. The normal alignment of the radius-lunate-capitate will be lost.

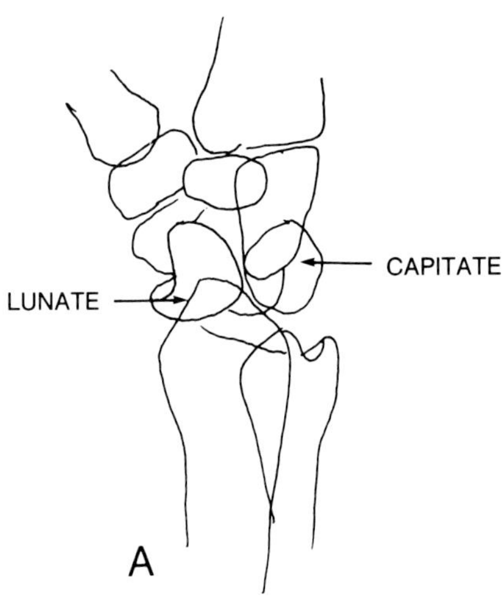

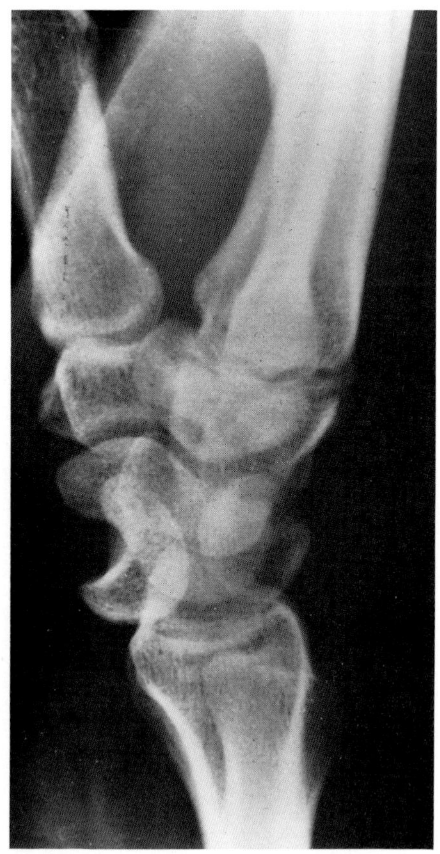

Fig. 7-13 (A) (Continues). A

Lunate Dislocations

The lunate dislocates anterior to the radius, but the remainder of the carpus is aligned with the radius (Fig. 7-13).

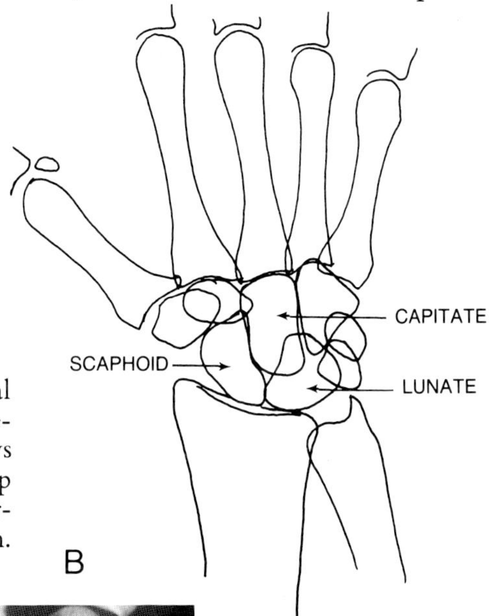

B

Fig. 7-13. Lunate dislocation. (A) Lateral view shows the lunate to be dislocated anterior to the wrist. (B) The AP view shows loss of the normal anatomical relationship of the carpal bones. The lunate is seen overlying the capitate, hamate, and triquetrium.

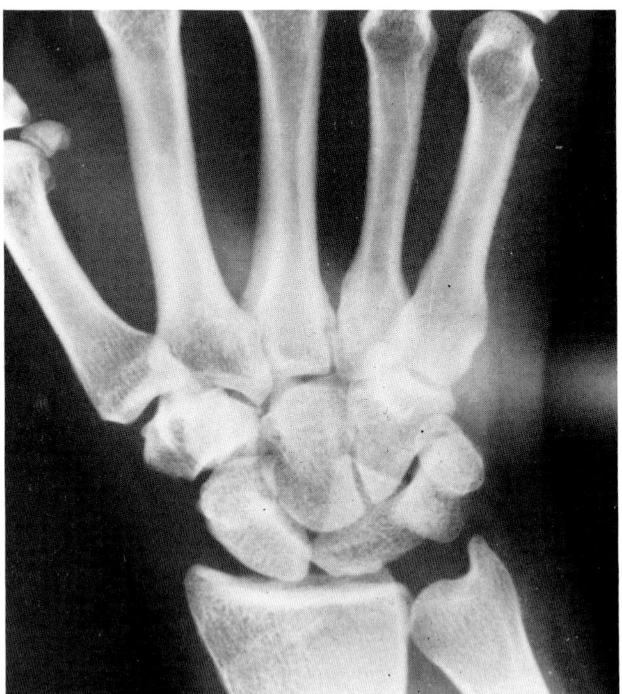

B

Perilunate Dislocations

The lunate remains aligned with the radius, and the remainder of the carpus is dislocated, usually dorsal to the lunate (Fig. 7-14). Usually, there is a concomitant fracture of the scaphoid, and the proximal portion of the scaphoid remains with the lunate while the distal portion dislocates with the carpus (trans-scaphoid perilunate dislocation).

COMPLICATIONS

Failure to recognize the complex nature of the dislocation.

TREATMENT

Closed reduction should be accomplished as quickly as possible. Open ligamentous repair or fracture fixation is usually required.

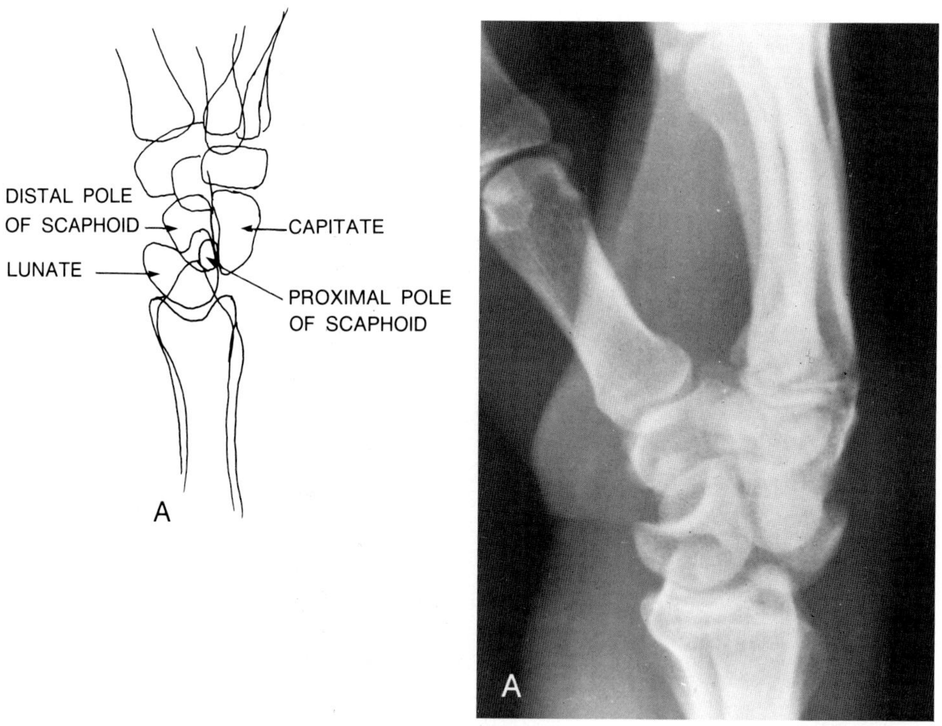

Fig. 7-14. Perilunate dislocation. (A) The lateral view reveals the lunate to be articulating with the radius but the remainder of the carpus is dislocated dorsally (Figure continues).

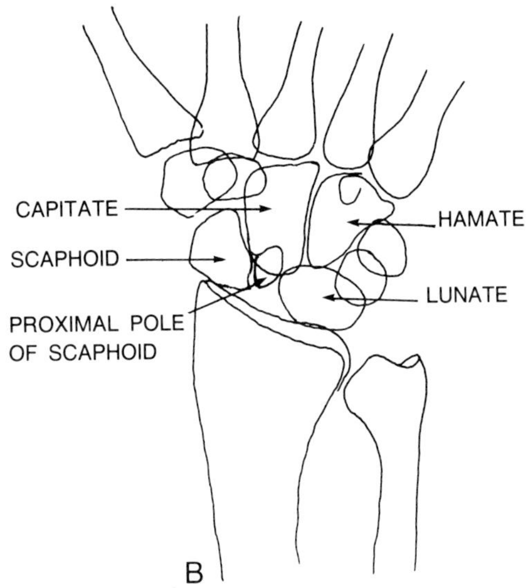

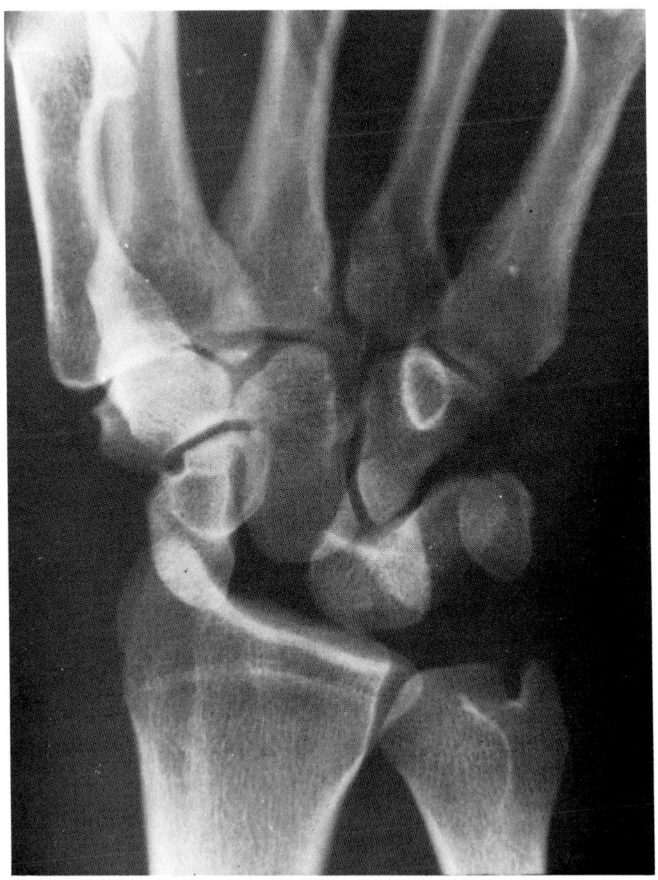

B

Fig. 7-14 (Continued). (B) AP view reveals the gross abnormality in the alignment of the carpus.

8 The Hand

The hand is the functional workhorse of the upper extremity. Through its diverse motions and functions, it is subject to a multitude of various stress, strains, and trauma. It is the object we often use to protect ourselves with, as well as to absorb the shock in "bracing" a fall. As a result, all the bones of the hand, as well as the joints, are subject to a variety of fractures and dislocations. The three basic radiographic views, AP (Fig. 8-1A), lateral (Fig. 8-1B), and oblique (Fig. 8-1C), will reveal the majority of hand injuries. When interested in a specific finger injury, it is best to get a radiograph of that specific finger for increased clarity and detail.

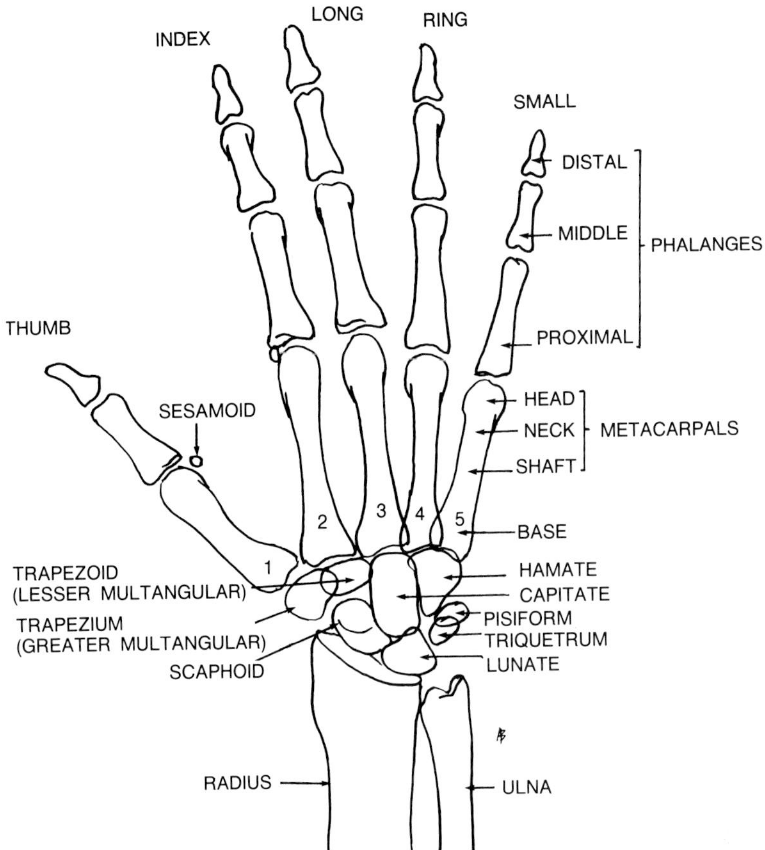

INDEX
LONG
RING
SMALL
DISTAL
MIDDLE
PROXIMAL
PHALANGES
THUMB
SESAMOID
HEAD
NECK
SHAFT
METACARPALS
1
2
3
4
5
BASE
TRAPEZOID
(LESSER MULTANGULAR)
TRAPEZIUM
(GREATER MULTANGULAR)
SCAPHOID
HAMATE
CAPITATE
PISIFORM
TRIQUETRUM
LUNATE
RADIUS
ULNA

A

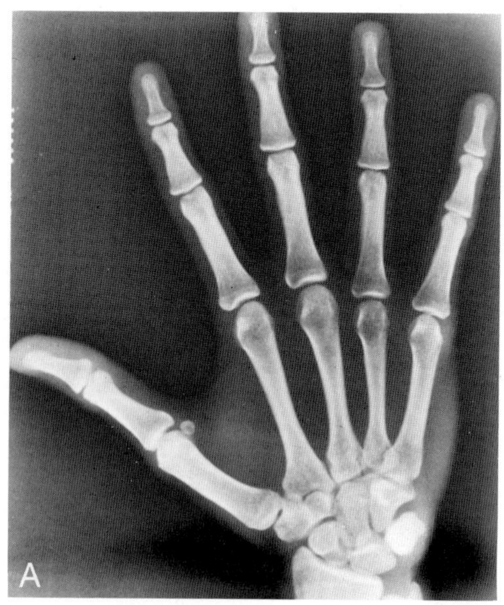

A

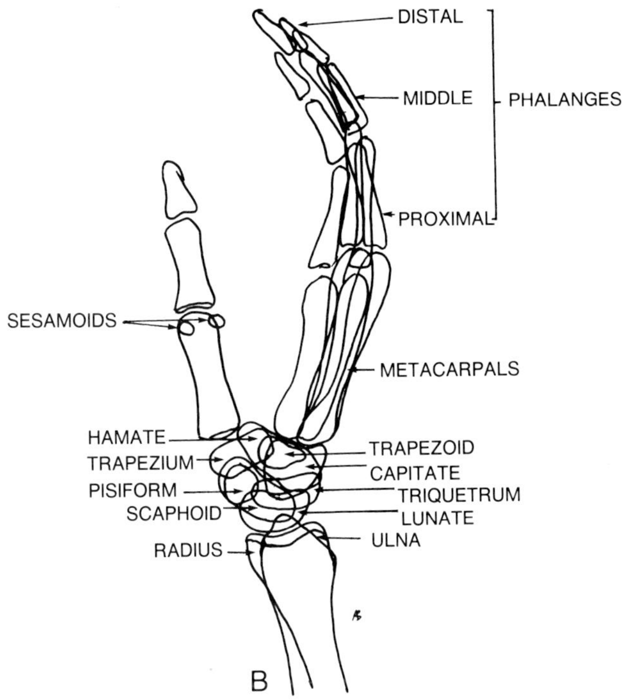

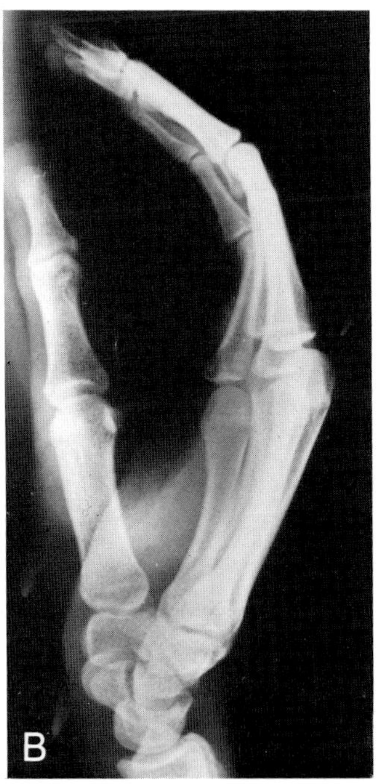

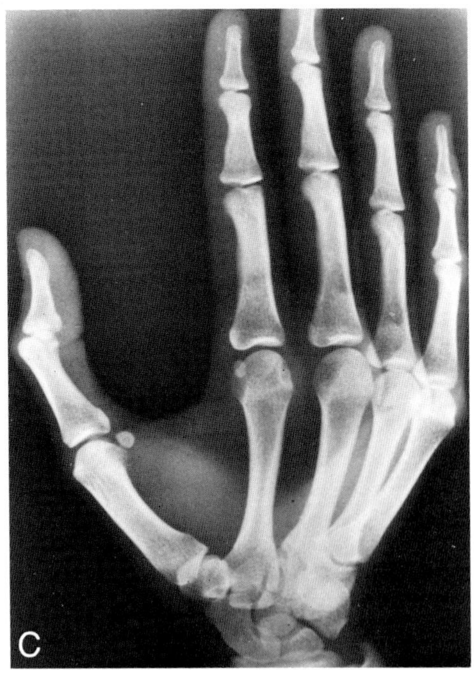

Fig. 8-1. (A) AP view of the hand — normal. (B) Lateral view of the hand — normal. (C) Oblique view of the hand — normal.

Fractures of the Metacarpals

The metacarpal is separated into four sections: the head, the neck, the shaft, and the base. The neck is the weakest area and a frequent site of fracture. The goal of treating metacarpal fractures is to restore alignment and rotation of the fingers.

MECHANISM

Fractures of the head are usually the result of a missile injury or a severe crush. Fractures of the neck are usually caused by a blow to the flexed metacarpal phalangeal joint, usually a punch. Fractures of the shaft are caused by a direct blow which creates a transverse of comminuted fracture, while torque of the fingers produces an oblique or spiral fracture. Fractures of the base have direct blows and crush injury as the most common etiologies.

CLINICAL PRESENTATION

There is pain and swelling of the hand with point tenderness at the site of the fracture. There may be shortening of the finger with loss of the "knuckle" when the fingers are flexed. The most important thing to assess is the alignment and rotation of the fingers (Fig. 8-2). A history of a fight is often obtained and a careful examination for a human bite to the hand should be made.

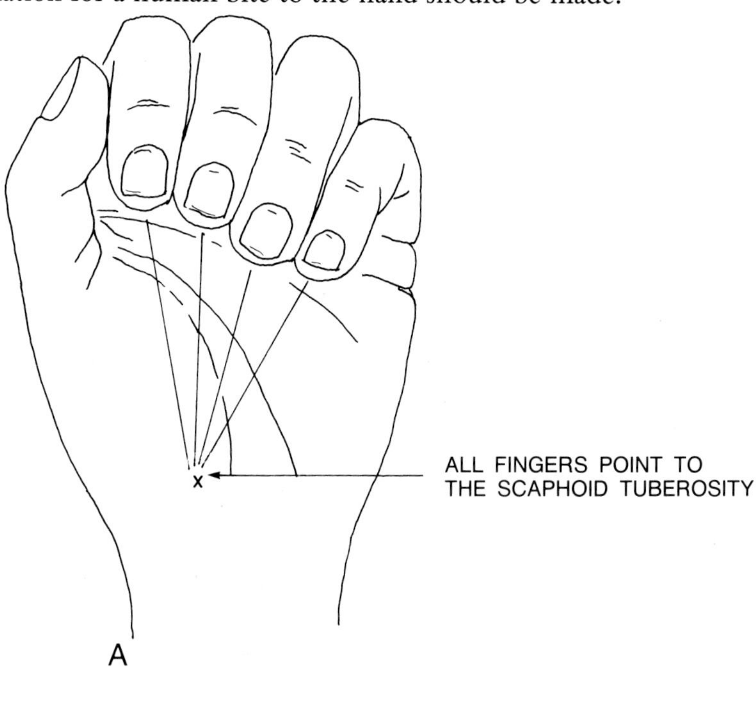

A

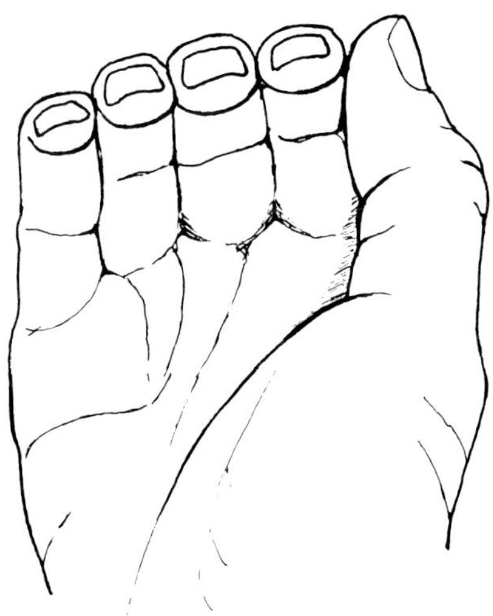

B

Fig. 8-2. (A) Normal hand-finger alignment. Note that a line drawn down the center of each finger points to the tuberosity of the navicular. Checking this relationship is an easy way to assess malrotation. (B) Note that when the fingers are held in a semiflexed position, there is a straight line formed by the nail and the tips of the fingers.

ROENTGENOGRAMS

AP, lateral, and oblique views (Fig. 8-3) are needed for full evaluation. However, it is the clinical examination which dictates the treatment in most cases. Fracture of the neck of the 5th metacarpal ("boxer's fracture") (Fig. 8-4) is the most common metacarpal fracture seen. It appears dorsally angulated. Transverse shaft fractures are inclined to angulate dorsally due to the deforming force of the intrinsic muscles. Oblique metacarpal shaft fractures may shorten or rotate.

COMPLICATIONS

Malunion or malalignment with rotation of any digit is unacceptable. More angulation of the metacarpal may be accepted in the ring and little fingers than in the long or index fingers. Stiffness occurs due to edema of the hand or immobilization with the metacarpophalangeal joints in extension. Carpometacarpal dislocation may not be appreciated. Any laceration or puncture over the metacarpophalangeal joint should be assumed to be a human bite and the wound left open.

TREATMENT

Closed reduction and placement in a hand dressing with a plaster splint and the metacarpophalangeal joints flexed to 70 degrees provides the best immobilization. If the digit is malaligned or rotated, open reduction and internal fixation may be necessary.

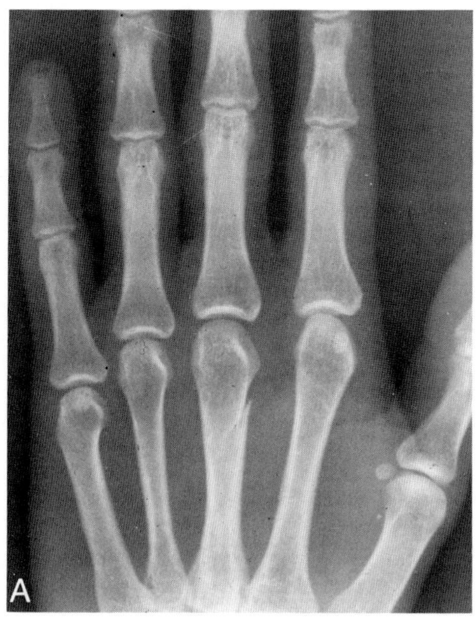

Fig. 8-3. (A) (Figure continues).

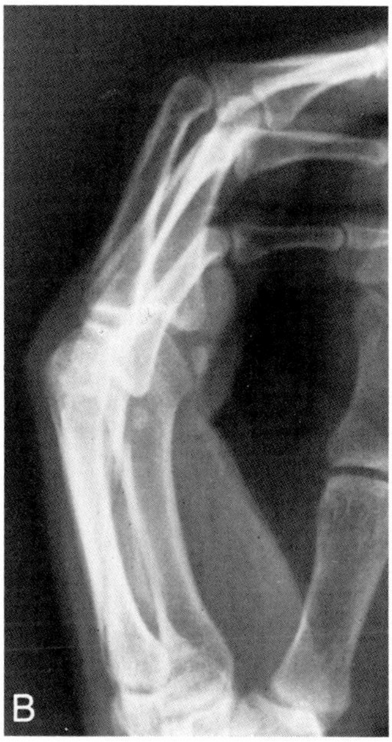

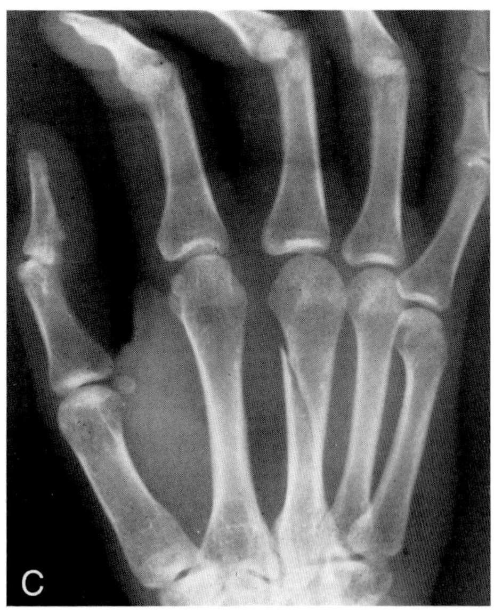

Fig. 8-3. Third metacarpal fracture. (A) AP view. (B) Lateral view. (C) Oblique view.

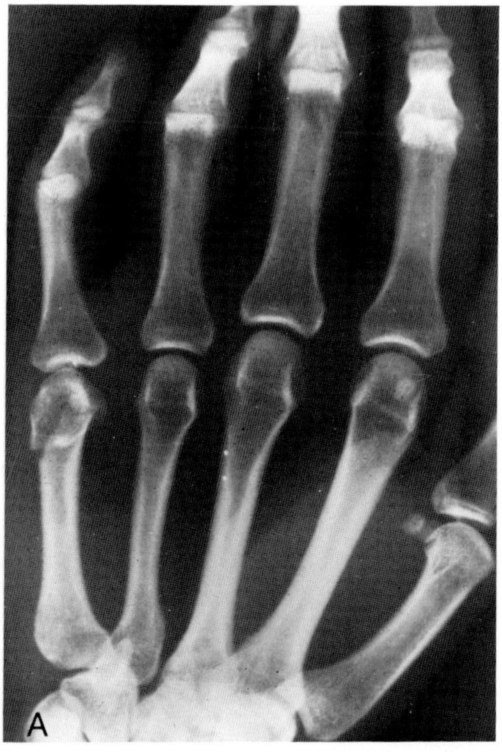

Fig. 8-4. (A) (Figure continues).

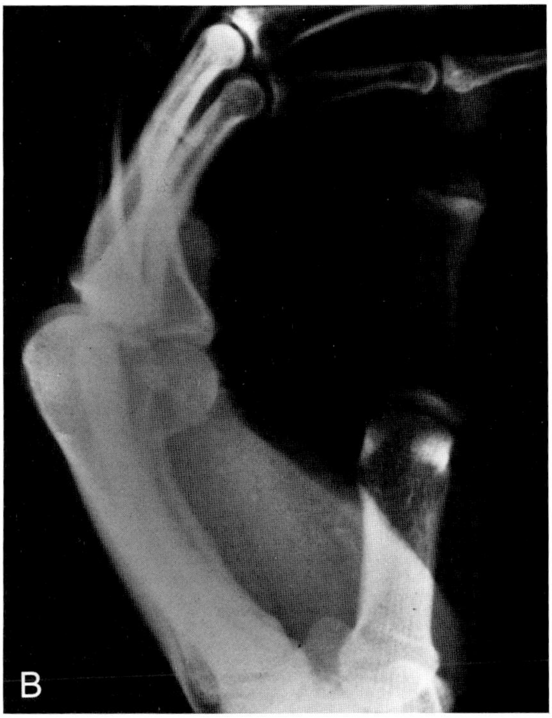

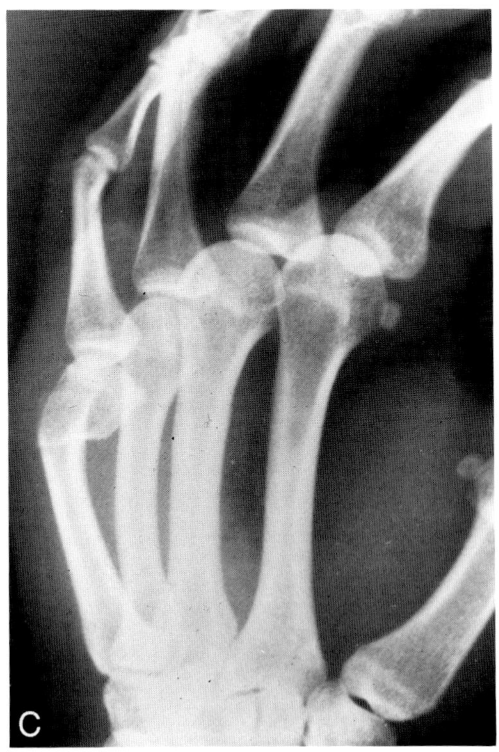

Fig. 8-4. Boxer's fracture — neck of the 5th metacarpal. (A) AP view. (B) Lateral view reveals the angulation. (C) Oblique view.

Bennett's Fracture Dislocation

This is an articular fracture of the first metacarpal base with radial subluxation of the metacarpal at the trapezio-metacarpal joint.

MECHANISM

An axial blow against a partially flexed metacarpal-phalangeal joint occurs, often in a fist fight.

CLINICAL PRESENTATION

There is pain and swelling of the hand with tenderness at the base of the first metacarpal. The thumb is shortened, and any motion is resisted secondary to pain.

ROENTGENOGRAMS

AP, lateral, and oblique views of the thumb (Fig. 8-5) demonstrate the displacement of this intra-articular fracture. A volar fragment is held to the trapezium while the rest of the metacarpal subluxates radially.

TREATMENT

Closed reduction may be attempted, but often is unsuccessful, and open reduction with internal fixation is needed.

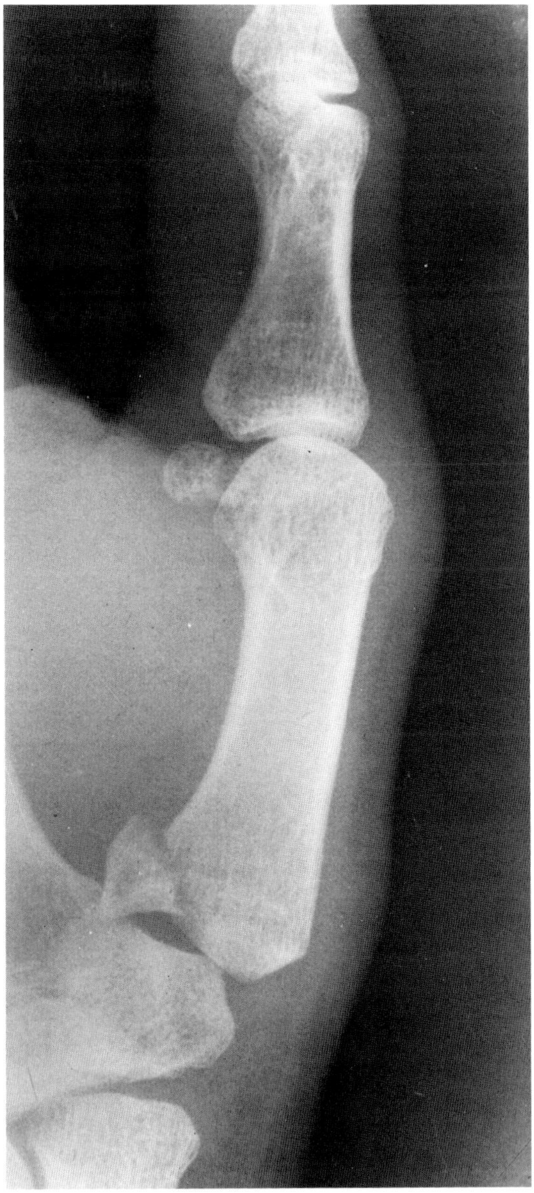

Fig. 8-5. Bennett's fracture dislocation of the thumb. The metacarpal fragment remains aligned to the trapezium while the thumb metacarpal subluxes radially due to muscular pull.

Rolando Fracture

This is a comminuted, intra-articular "T" or "Y" fracture of the base of the first metacarpal. There are dorsal and volar articular fragments which make internal fixation necessary. Skeletal traction with early motion is useful in the very comminuted fractures.

Extra-Articular First Metacarpal Fractures

These fractures result from a similar mechanism to the Bennett's fracture, but with slightly different stresses. Closed reduction in a thumb spica for immobilization is usually satisfactory (Fig. 8-6).

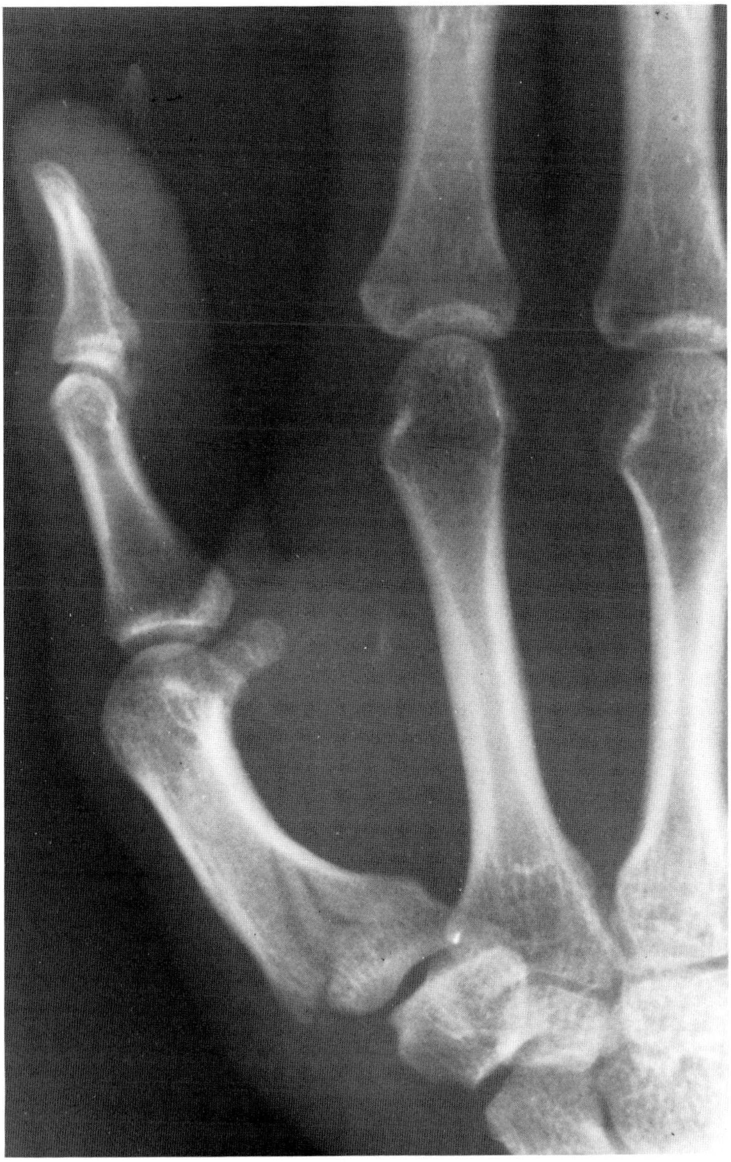

Fig. 8-6. Extra-articular fracture of the thumb metacarpal.

Gamekeeper's Thumb

This is an injury to the ulnar collateral ligament of the metacarpal-phalangeal joint which produces weakness or loss of stability in pinch.

MECHANISM

A valgus or radial stress to the metacarpal-phalangeal joint of the thumb tears the ulnar collateral ligament. Catching the thumb on a ski pole or similar object is a common history.

CLINICAL PRESENTATION

Swelling and tenderness on the ulnar side of the thumb metacarpal-phalangeal joint is present. The stability of the joint should be tested.

ROENTGENOGRAMS

AP, lateral, and oblique views (Fig. 8-7) of the thumb can be normal, or a small avulsion of the proximal phalanx may be seen. A stress roentgenogram (a true AP of the *thumb*) under anesthesia will help to document the stability of the joint.

COMPLICATIONS

Chronic instability is the rule if the injury is not recognized and treated.

TREATMENT

Placement in a thumb spica cast is the treatment for incomplete tears, but complete tears should be repaired operatively. Displaced avulsion fractures may need internal fixation.

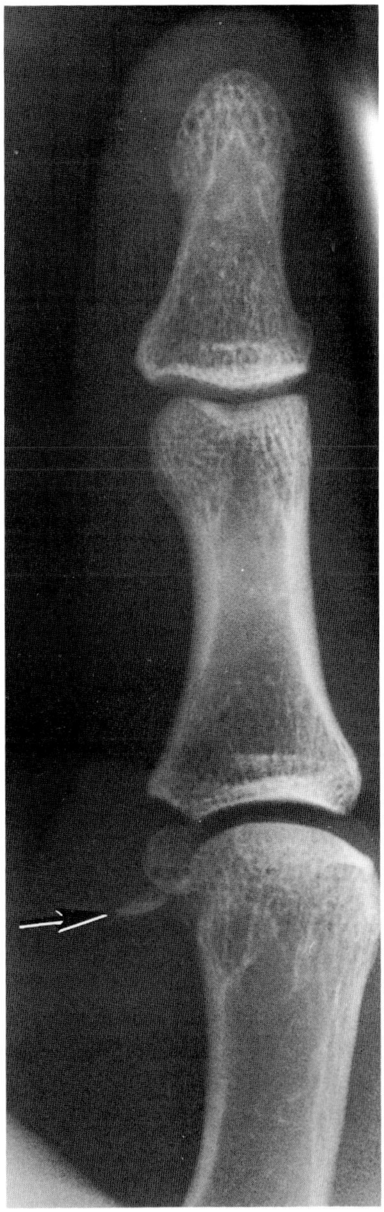

Fig. 8-7. Gamekeeper's thumb. The ulnar collateral ligament has avulsed a piece of bone from the proximal phalanx (arrow).

PHALANGES

Finger alignment is the goal. Displacement, rotation, angulation, the mechanism of injury, and the deforming forces must be assessed and corrected to achieve the best results.

Distal Phalanx Injuries

Fifty percent of hand fractures occur in the distal phalanx. Two specific injuries will be discussed separately.

MECHANISM

Crushing injury is the common mechanism, but several types of fracture can result: longitudinal, transverse, or comminuted.

CLINICAL PRESENTATION

Severe soft tissue and nail injuries may be more disabling than the fracture. The distal tuft is swollen and very tender. If the nail is intact, a subungal hematoma is often present and very painful. These fractures are often open.

ROENTGENOGRAMS

AP, lateral, and oblique views (Fig. 8-8) of the involved *finger* should be obtained, not films of the hand.

TREATMENT

Sterile drainage of the subungal hematoma will reduce pain. Debridement of an open wound is necessary. The finger should be aligned and splinted to protect it and to relieve pain. It is essential to secure the splint with stretchable material, which allows for swelling. An acutely injured finger should not be taped to a splint. Maximum immobilization and protection can be given with a full hand dressing, including plaster.

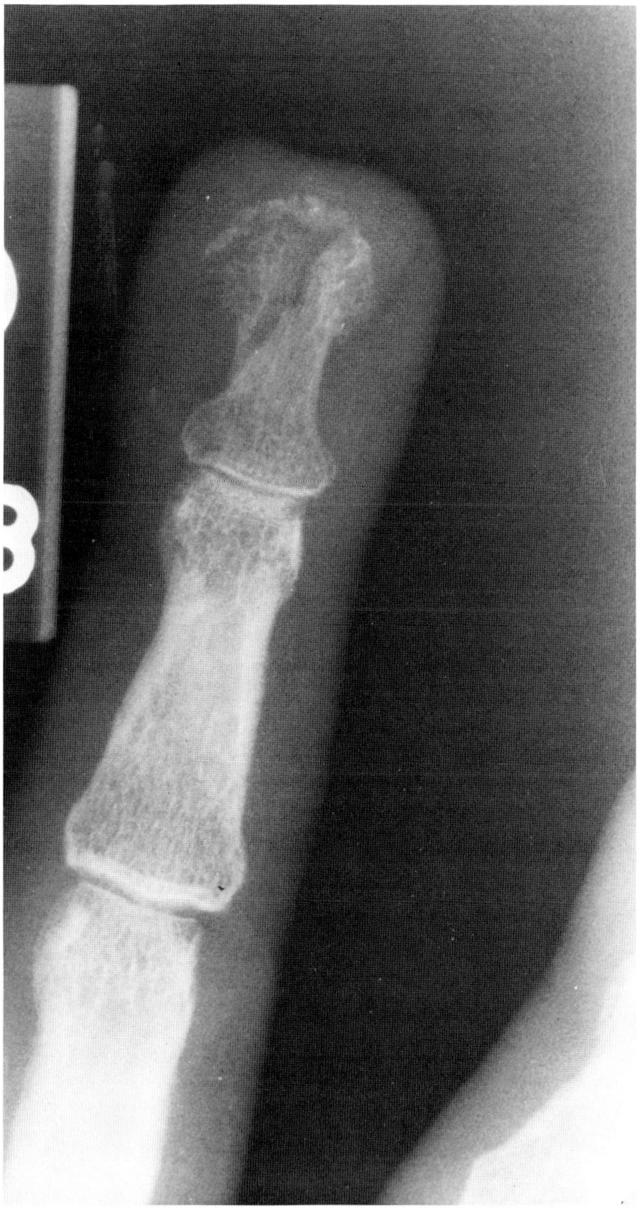

Fig. 8-8. Distal phalanx fracture. This is a crushing injury to the distal phalanx.

Mallet Finger

MECHANISM AND CLINICAL PRESENTATION

This injury results from forcible flexion of the extended DIP joint. Three different problems present with the same injury:

1. Loss of extensor tendon continuity without a fracture. There can be a frank rupture of the tendon or mere stretching. The patient is unable to extend the DIP joint fully.
2. A small, dorsal avulsion fracture of the proximal aspect of the distal phalanx at the extensor insertion.
3. Intra-articular fracture of the distal phalanx, which includes the extensor insertion.

Each type of injury will result in inability to extend the DIP joint fully.

ROENTGENOGRAMS

AP and lateral of the finger (Fig. 8-9) show the lesion and the extent of articular surface involved.

TREATMENT

Splint the DIP joint in full extension.

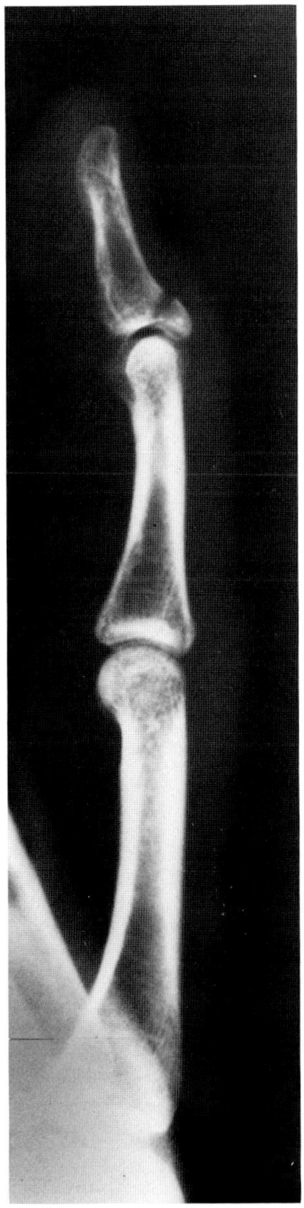

Fig. 8-9. Mallet finger fracture. This injury is an avulsion fracture caused by the pull of the extensor tendon.

Volar Avulsion

MECHANISM

This injury may be due to forceful extension of the flexed finger or resisted flexion of the DIP joint, causing avulsion of the bony insertion of the flexor digitorum profundus tendon.

CLINICAL PRESENTATION

This injury presents with pain and swelling at the DIP joint without any obvious deformity. Testing the finger will show the loss of DIP flexion.

ROENTGENOGRAMS

AP, lateral, and oblique views (Fig. 8-10) reveal the position and size of the avulsed fragment with most information being found on the lateral film.

COMPLICATIONS

The injury may be overlooked with a small fracture if DIP flexion is not tested. This lesion is commonly missed.

TREATMENT

Open reduction is necessary to restore tendon continuity.

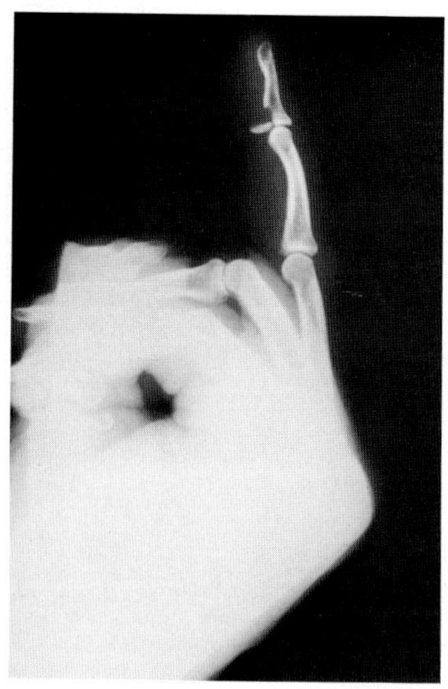

Fig. 8-10. Profundus avulsion fracture. This injury occurs at the insertion of the flexor profundus tendon into the distal phalanx.

Middle Phalanx

MECHANISM

This fracture usually results from a blow to the hand or a crush injury. The relationship to the insertion of the superficialis tendon is the determinant of the deformity.

CLINICAL PRESENTATION

There is pain and swelling of the finger at the middle phalanx with angulation of the fracture. If the fracture is proximal to the superficialis tendon insertion, there is volar angulation; dorsal angulation occurs if the fracture is distal to the insertion of the superficialis tendon.

TREATMENT

Reduction and alignment of the finger is needed. Placement in a hand dressing is the ideal immobilization.

Proximal Phalanx Injuries

This phalanx is injured more often than the middle, but less often than the distal phalanx.

MECHANISM

These, as with most hand fractures, can result from torsion or a direct blow to the finger.

CLINICAL PRESENTATION

The proximal segment of the finger is painful and swollen. Finger rotation and alignment can be normal. Transverse fractures usually angulate volarly.

ROENTGENOGRAMS

AP and lateral views (Fig. 8-11) of the finger are necessary.

TREATMENT

Reduction and alignment of the finger. A hand dressing is probably the best immobilization.

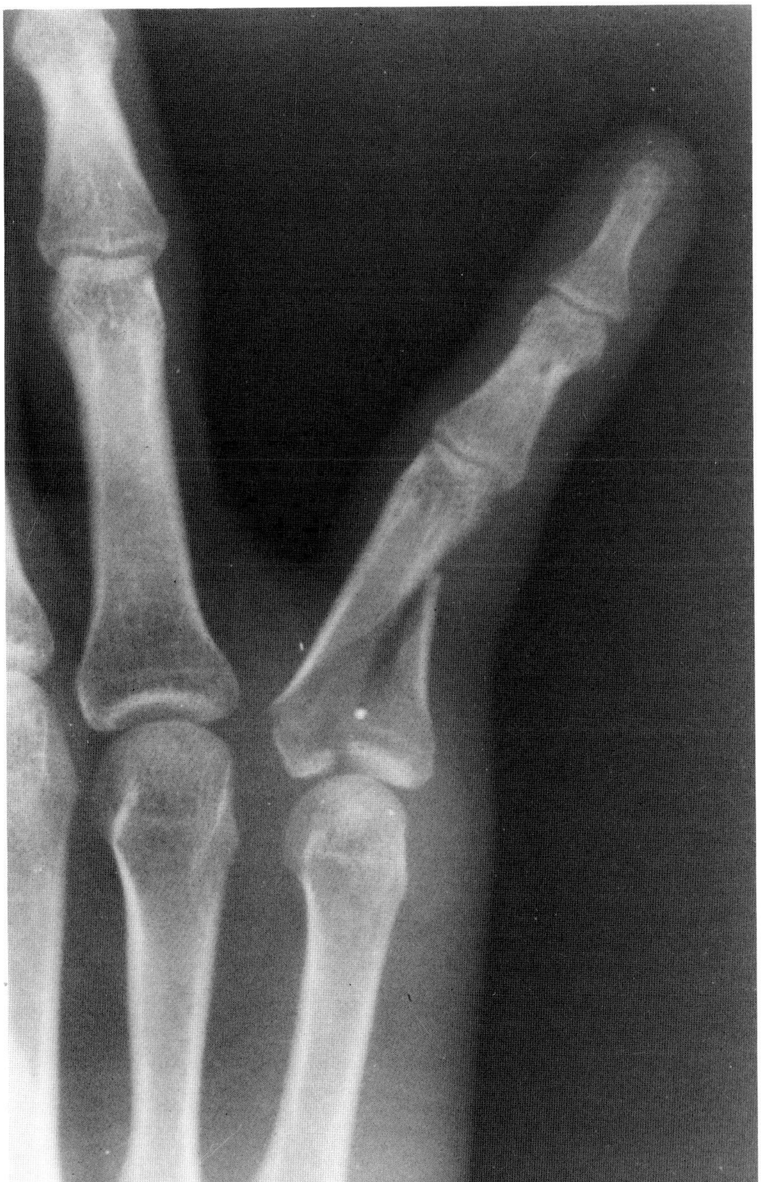

Fig. 8-11. Proximal phalanx fracture. Note that this fracture does go intra-articular in this particular patient.

Metacarpophalangeal Dislocations

Dislocations result from a fall on the outstretched hand with hyperextension of the MP joint and dorsal dislocation.

CLINICAL PRESENTATION

Most commonly, these dislocations occur in the index or little finger. There is a swelling and prominence dorsally. Puckering of the proximal palmar crease is pathognomonic of an "irreducible" MP dislocation.

ROENTGENOGRAMS

AP, lateral, and oblique views of the hand (Fig. 8-12) will reveal the dorsal dislocation and demonstrate any concomitant fractures. The phalanx may be at 90 degrees to the metacarpal in a simple dislocation. Widening of the joint space may be a clue that soft tissue is interposed into the joint with the irreducible-type, and the phalanx will be parallel to the metacarpal in this complex dislocation.

COMPLICATIONS

Soft tissue interposition may make closed reduction impossible.

TREATMENT

Closed reduction is easy for the simple dislocation but may be impossible in the complex variety.

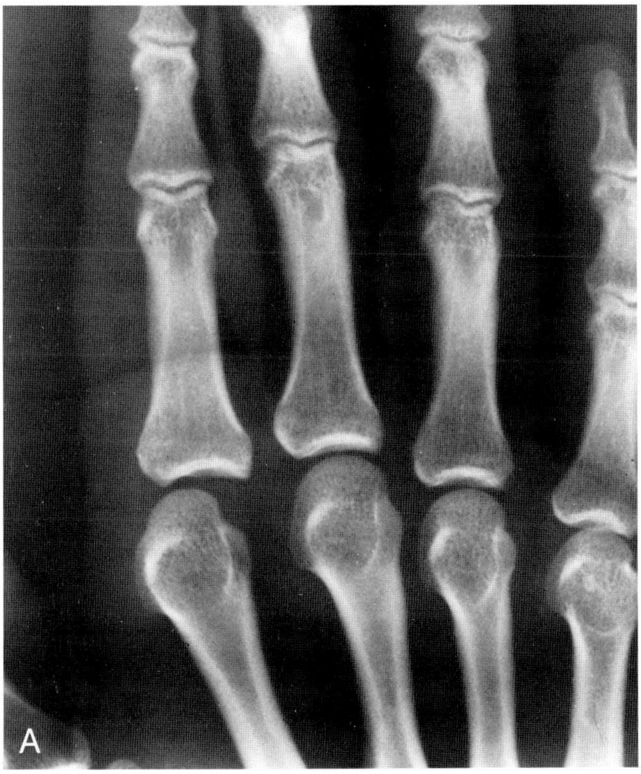

Fig. 8-12 (A). (Figure continues).

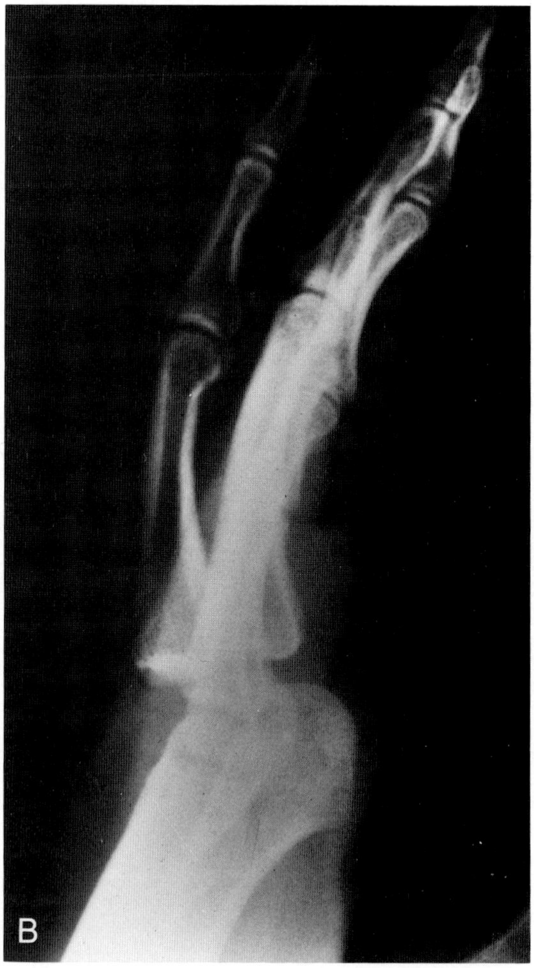

Fig. 8-12 (B) (Figure continues).

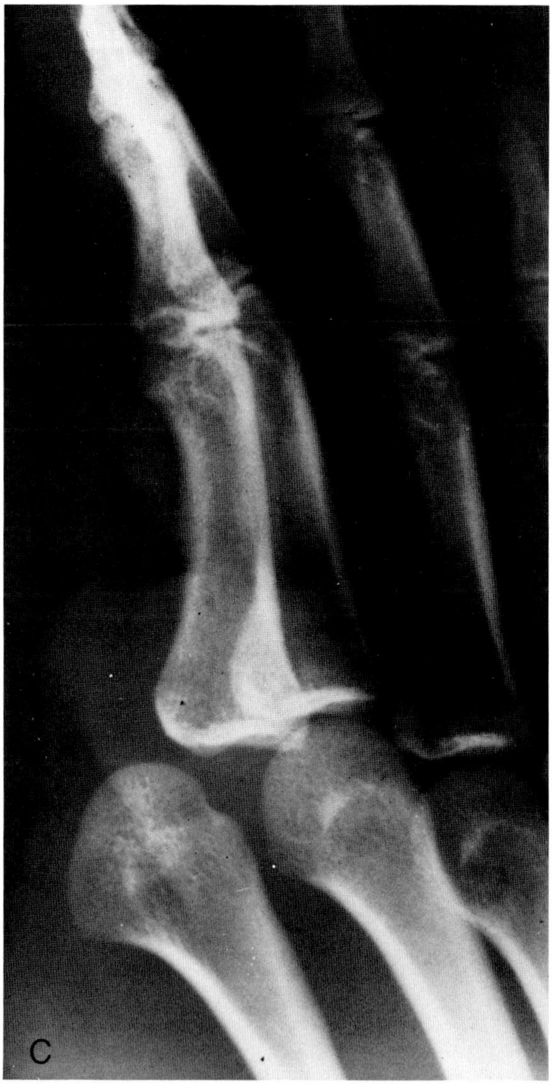

Fig. 8-12 (Continued). Metacarpophalangeal dislocation. (A) AP view reveals a slight abnormality in the contour of the index finger MP joint. (B) Lateral view reveals the index finger to be dislocated dorsally at the MP joint. (C) Oblique view.

INTERPHALANGEAL DISLOCATIONS

Dislocation of the PIP joint is more common than the DIP joint. Dorsal dislocation is much more common than volar dislocation.

Dorsal Dislocation

MECHANISM

These dislocations occur from hyperextension with rupture of the volar plate.

CLINICAL PRESENTATION

There is gross deformity with pain and swelling of the IP joint in the finger.

ROENTGENOGRAMS

AP and lateral views (Fig. 8-13) of the finger should be obtained before and after reduction to preclude any associated fracture.

COMPLICATIONS

Soft tissue interposition may make closed reduction impossible.

TREATMENT

These dislocations are reduced with longitudinal traction. The hand and fingers should be immobilized.

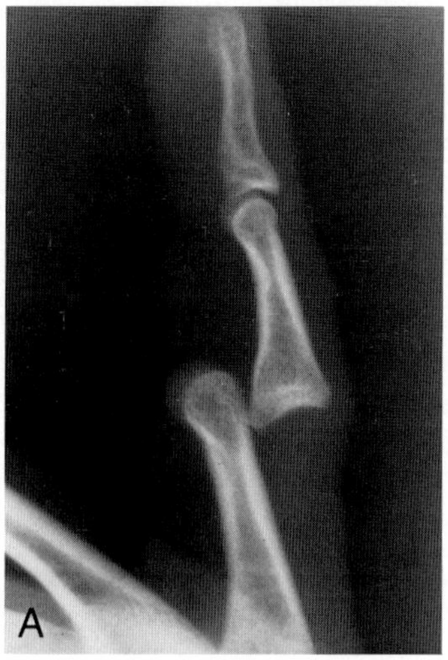

Fig. 8-13 (A) (Figure continues).

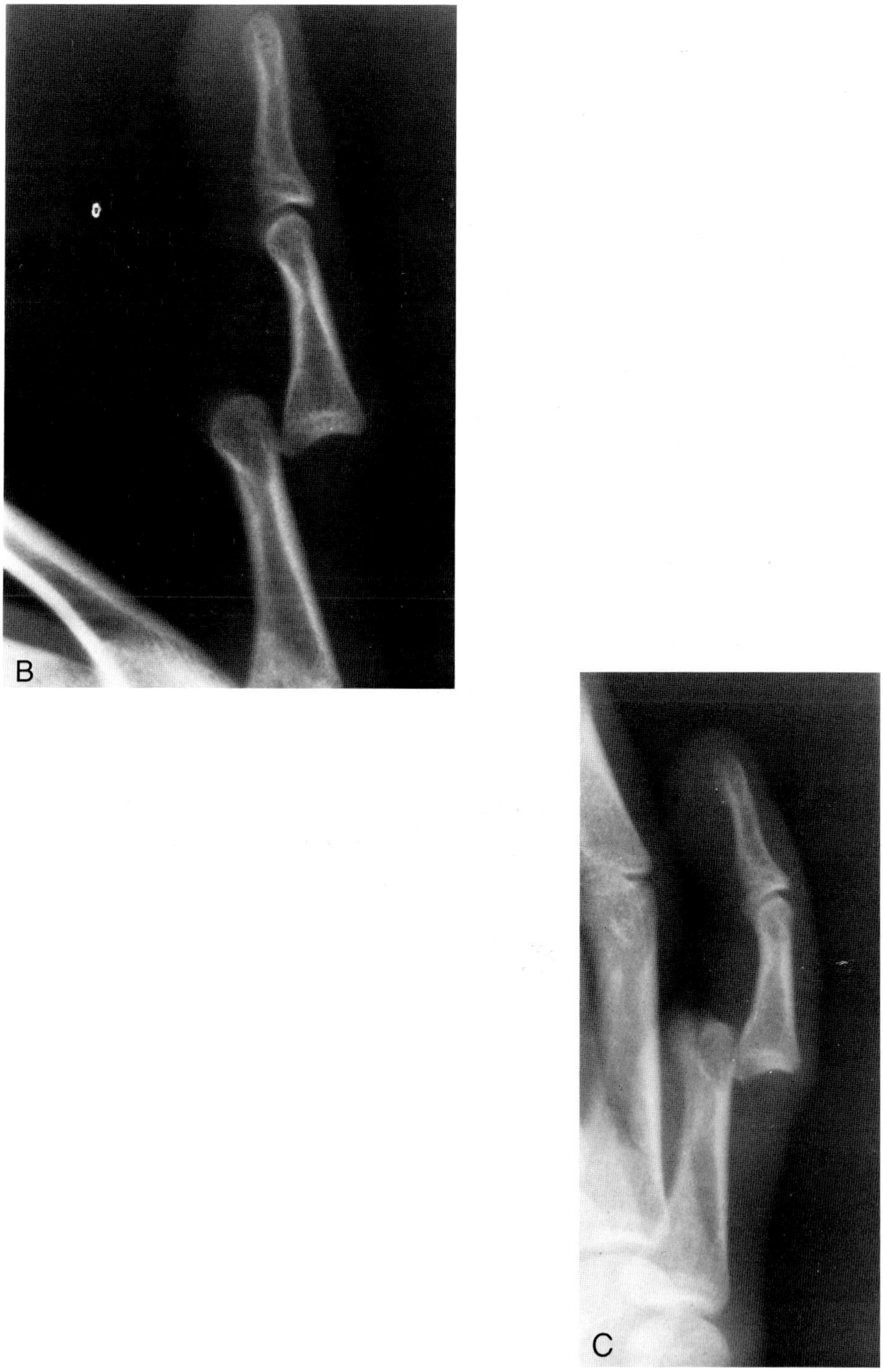

Fig. 8-13 (Continued). PIP dislocation. (A) AP view. (B) Lateral view reveals dorsal dislocation. (C) Oblique view.

Volar Dislocations

MECHANISM

The force is directed anteriorly or volarly against the finger but there may be torsional forces as well, with associated rupture of the extensor mechanism and herniation of the phalanx through the extensor.

CLINICAL PRESENTATION

There is gross deformity with pain and swelling of the IP joint.

ROENTGENOGRAMS

AP and lateral views, before and after reduction (Fig. 8-14) are needed to define any associated fractures.

COMPLICATIONS

Soft tissue interposition may make closed reduction impossible.

TREATMENT

Reduction with longitudinal traction. Immobilize the IP joint in full extension; the MP joint should be flexed 70 degrees. Some authors feel immediate repair of the extensor mechanism is required.

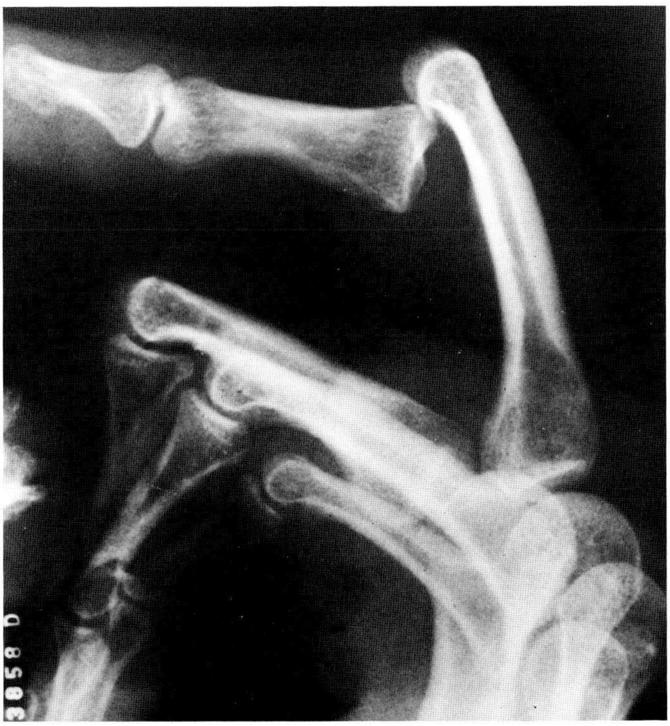

Fig. 8-14. Volar PIP dislocation. This rare injury is best seen on the lateral view.

PART III

The Lower Extremities

Larry S. Eisenfeld
Randall J. Lewis

9 The Pelvis

The bony pelvis serves to protect the pelvic/abdominal viscera, and serves as a site of origin for many of the muscles of the lower extremities. Injuries to the pelvis usually result from motor vehicle accidents or falls in the elderly. The routine AP view of the pelvis (Fig. 9-1) will reveal most fractures. In patients with significantly displaced pelvic fractures, one must be concerned about visceral injuries and severe hemorrhage.

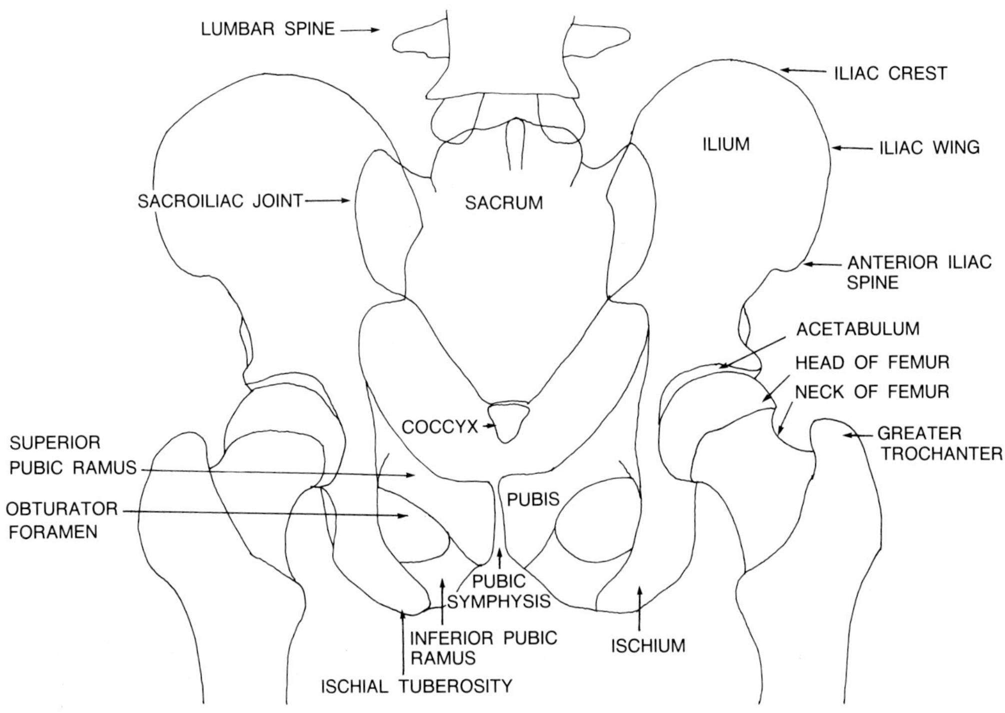

Fig. 9-1. AP view of the pelvis — normal.

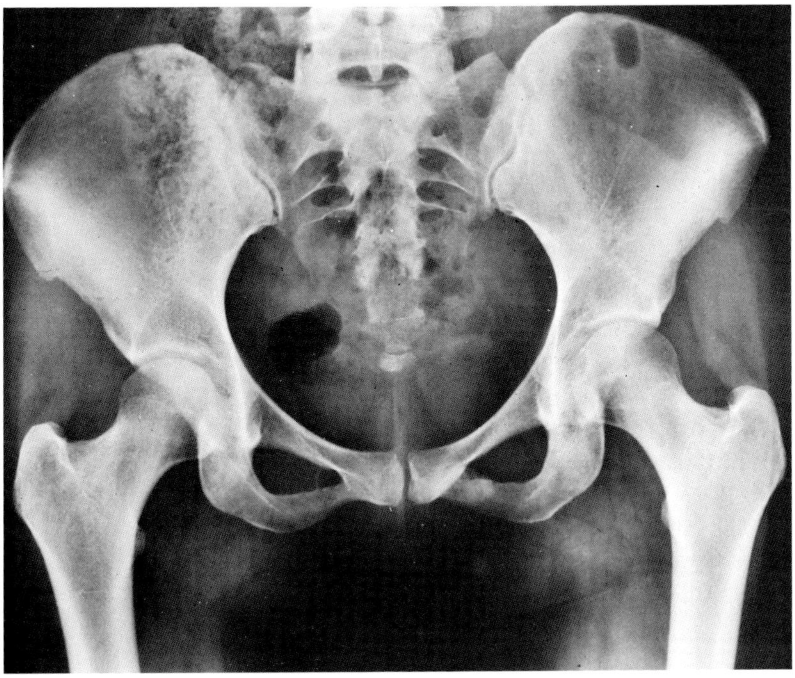

Fig. 9-1. (Continued).

Pelvic Fractures

MECHANISM

High velocity trauma (motor vehicle accidents) or falls in the elderly.

CLINICAL PRESENTATION

The patient complains of pain and tenderness at the fracture site. Injuries are often minor, but may be severe in the multiple trauma patient. The physician should check the pelvis for stability and examine the abdomen for associated injuries.

ROENTGENOGRAMS

The AP roentgenogram of the pelvis (Figs. 9-1, 9-2) is satisfactory for delineation of most pelvic fractures; additional studies (oblique views; tomograms) are usually not required in the emergency room.

COMPLICATIONS

Life-threatening associated injuries are frequent in high energy trauma. Severe retroperitoneal hemorrhage occurs in forty percent of cases. Visceral damage most often involves the urinary tract. Rupture of the urethra occurs in 8 to 10 percent of patients and bladder rupture in 4 percent, most often in males. Gynecologic and intestinal injury is less common. Neurologic injury may occur due to nerve root stretch, cauda equina injury, or direct peripheral nerve injury. Concomitant musculoskeletal injuries, such as hip fracture, hip dislocation, patella fracture, and Lisfranc dislocation are common.

TREATMENT

All patients with pelvic fractures should have intravenous fluids, urinalysis, abdominal and hip roentgenograms, and be crossmatched for blood. Life-threatening injury to the head, chest, and abdomen must be excluded. Treatment of the pelvic fracture depends on the nature of the disruption and the preference of the treating surgeon.

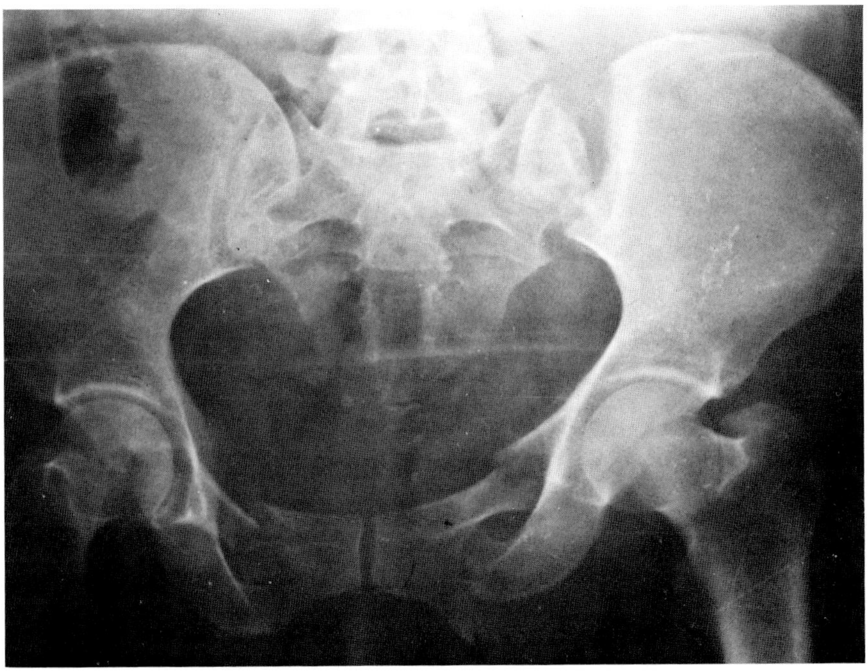

Fig. 9-2. Complex pelvic fracture, involving the iliac wing and both superior and inferior pubic rami. A high incidence of visceral injuries is associated with this fracture.

Complex Pelvic Fractures

Complex pelvic fractures involve two breaks in the pelvic ring and are unstable. There is a high incidence of associated injuries.

MECHANISM

High velocity injury — either severe falls or motor vehicle accidents.

CLINICAL PRESENTATION

Unstable pelvic fractures usually occur in multiple trauma victims. Life-threatening blood loss is frequent and must not be overlooked while treating other obvious injuries. Pelvic stability is evaluated with anterior pressure over the iliac spine or lateral compressive forces applied to the iliac wings. Crepitus and grating may be felt and an "open book" may be appreciated when pressing on the iliac spines.

ROENTGENOGRAMS

An AP view of the pelvis (Fig. 9-2) reveals the fracture. Further evaluation may be needed (oblique views, tomograms, CAT scans) once the patient has been stabilized.

COMPLICATIONS

There is a high incidence of associated injuries. It is essential to evaluate the hips, abdomen, chest, and head. Significant blood loss is the rule, and may be life-threatening.

TREATMENT

Immediate resuscitation with intravenous fluids and blood. Stabilization in a pelvic sling, traction, or an external fixation device may be appropriate. Bedrest is often satisfactory treatment.

Pubic Ramus Fractures

Fractures of the pubic rami account for one-third of all pelvic fractures.

MECHANISM

The isolated pubic ramus fracture is most often seen in elderly patients after minor trauma, such as a fall.

CLINICAL PRESENTATION

Pain over the pubic ramus and with hip motion. A ramus fracture does not interrupt the integrity of the pelvic ring and is stable.

ROENTGENOGRAMS

An AP view of the pelvis will reveal the fracture (Fig. 9-3).

COMPLICATIONS

There is a high association of hip fractures, other pelvic fractures, and visceral injury in high velocity injuries.

TREATMENT

Treatment is symptomatic, consisting of bedrest and progressive ambulation with weight-bearing as tolerated.

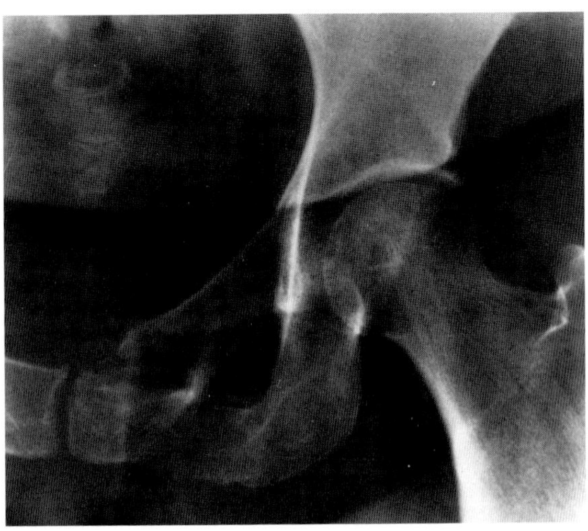

Fig. 9-3. Pubic ramus fracture. Note fracture of both the inferior and superior pubic rami.

ACETABULUM

The acetabulum is the socket portion of the hip joint. There are two common types of acetabular injury.

Posterior Fracture-Dislocation of the Hip

MECHANISM

Occurs most commonly in a motor vehicle accident. With the hip in the flexed position, the knee strikes the dashboard. The femur is driven posteriorly, causing fracture of the posterior wall of the acetabulum and posterior dislocation of the hip.

CLINICAL PRESENTATION

The leg is shortened and held in internal rotation. The neurovascular status must be carefully evaluated due to the high incidence of associated sciatic and peroneal nerve injury.

ROENTGENOGRAMS

An AP view of the hip will reveal the injury (Fig. 9-4). The femoral head is seen overlying the acetabulum instead of being concentric with the socket. Shenton's line is disrupted and the femur is held in internal rotation. Fragments of the posterior lip of the acetabulum may or may not be visualized on routine films. The dislocated femoral head may appear smaller in size, as it is closer to the radiographic plate. After reduction of the hip is achieved, tomograms, CAT scan, or oblique roentgenograms may be necessary to help delineate the size and displacement of the fragments.

COMPLICATIONS

Sciatic or peroneal nerve injury occurs in almost 20 percent. There is a high incidence of late, post-traumatic arthritis and aseptic necrosis of the femoral head following a fracture-dislocation. Venous thrombosis and pulmonary embolism are always significant risks following pelvic injury.

TREATMENT

Reduction as soon as possible. This usually requires general anesthesia.

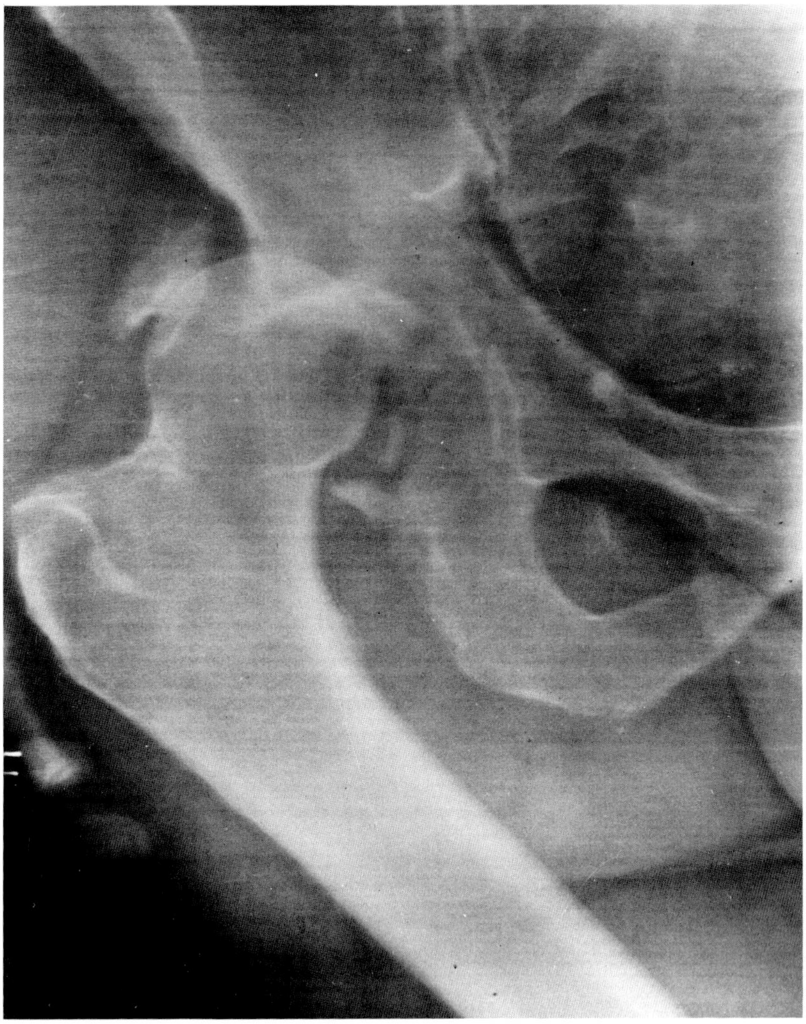

Fig. 9-4. Posterior fracture-dislocation of the hip.

Central Fracture of the Acetabulum

MECHANISM

This injury results from a force translated along the shaft of the femur with the hip held in the extended position. The forces are transmitted centrally and superiorly, producing a central fracture-dislocation, with displacement of the head of the femur into the pelvis.

CLINICAL PRESENTATION

The leg appears shortened. Neurovascular injuries are less common. Motion of the hip is severely restricted and resisted because of pain.

ROENTGENOGRAMS

An AP view of the pelvis (Fig. 9-5) reveals the injury. Oblique views, tomograms, and CAT scans may be indicated on a non-emergency basis for further evaluation.

COMPLICATIONS

Femoral neck fracture and pubic rami fractures are common. If the fracture involves the superior "weight-bearing dome" of the acetabulum the prognosis is poorer, as late degenerative arthritis may ensue.

TREATMENT

Reduction of the hip should be achieved as soon as possible. Skeletal traction helps to stabilize the fracture fragments and control bleeding.

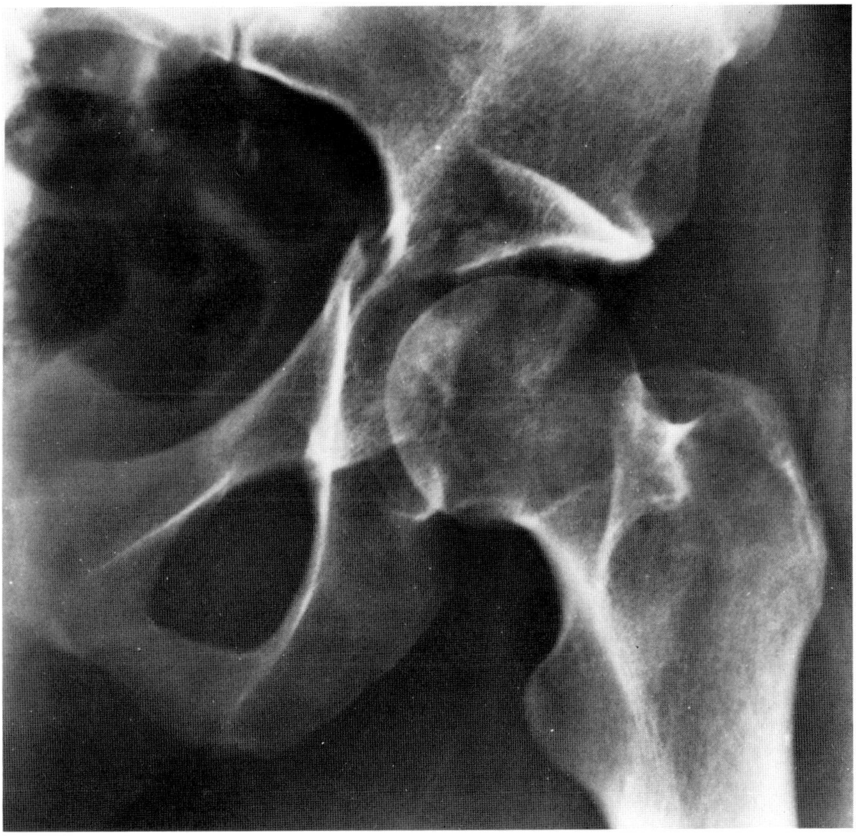

Fig. 9-5. Central acetabular fracture.

10 The Hip and Femur

Most hip fractures occur in the elderly with minor trauma. Hip fractures can be divided into two types: intracapsular and extracapsular. Each type entails a different treatment, prognosis, and different complications. The routine views necessary in the Emergency Room are the AP view (Fig. 10-1A) and a lateral view (Fig. 10-1B).

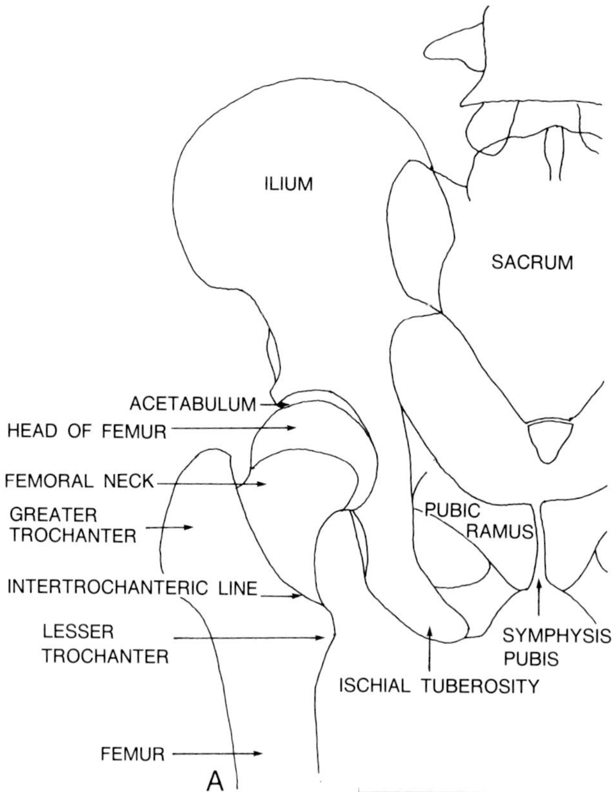
ILIUM
SACRUM
ACETABULUM
HEAD OF FEMUR
FEMORAL NECK
GREATER
TROCHANTER
INTERTROCHANTERIC LINE
LESSER
TROCHANTER
PUBIC
RAMUS
SYMPHYSIS
PUBIS
ISCHIAL TUBEROSITY
FEMUR
A

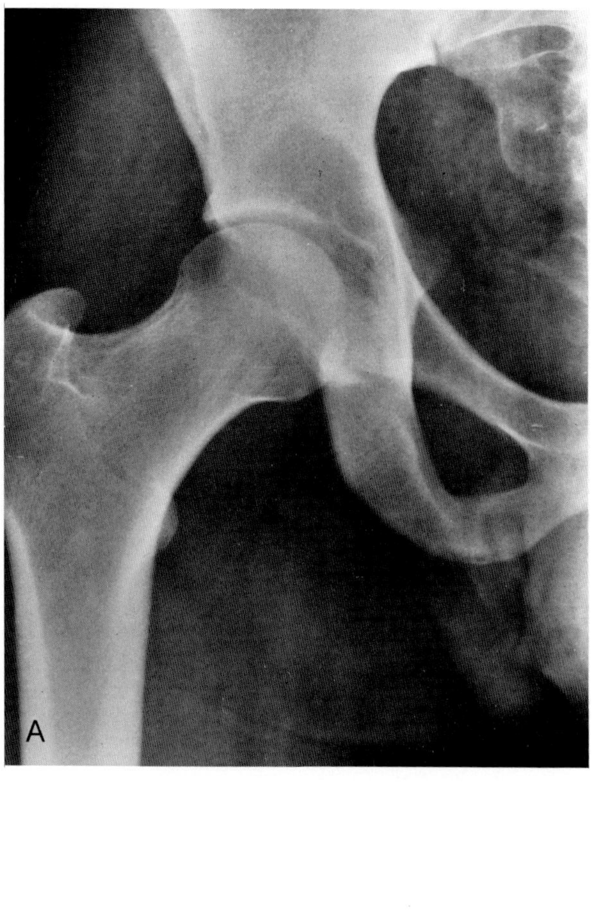
A

Fig. 10-1 (A).

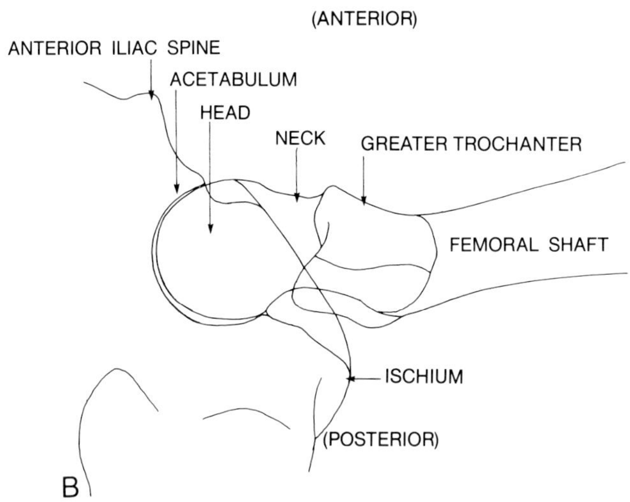

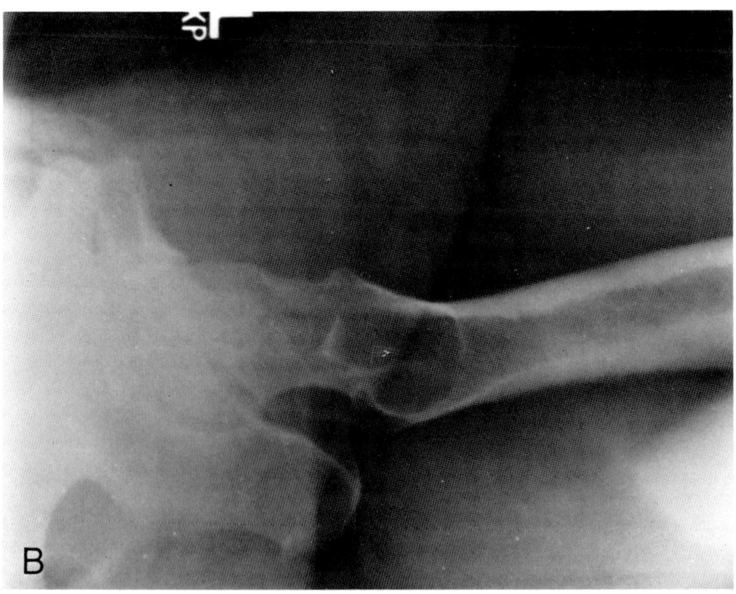

Fig. 10-1. (A) AP view of the hip (normal). (B) Lateral view of the hip (normal).

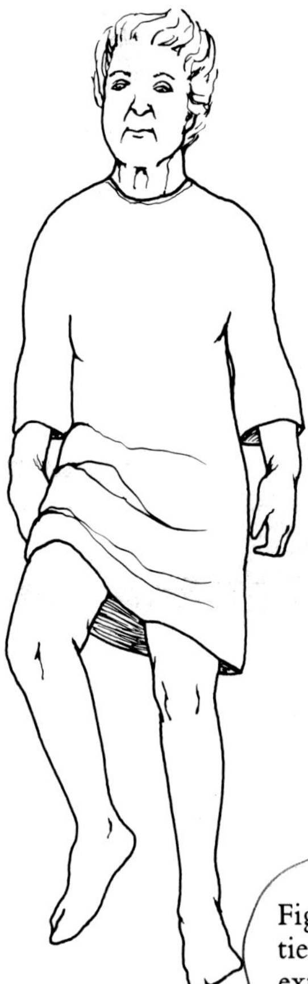

Fig. 10-2. The "classical" position assumed by patients with a hip fracture. The leg is shortened and externally rotated.

Intracapsular or Femoral Neck Fractures

MECHANISM

Usually a fall in elderly patients. High energy trauma in young adults.

CLINICAL PRESENTATION

The patient with an impacted fracture may complain of groin or hip pain. There may be a decreased range of motion, but no deformity. He or she may even be able to ambulate. Patients with displaced fractures are unable to walk; the leg appears shortened and rotated (Fig. 10-2). Any elderly patient who complains of hip pain or inability to walk after a fall should be assumed to have a hip fracture until proven otherwise.

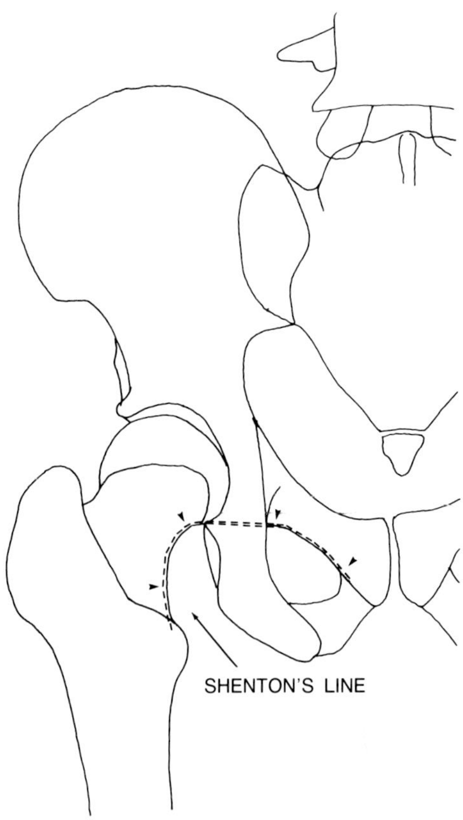

Fig. 10-3. Shenton's line. A line drawn along the medial margin of the femoral neck should continue in a smooth arc along the lower border of the superior pubic ramus. A disruption of the arc represents some pathology within the hip, either a fracture or a dislocation.

ROENTGENOGRAMS

In displaced fractures, the AP roentgenograms (Fig. 10-4A) will reveal a disruption of Shenton's line (Fig. 10-3). A lateral roentgenogram (Fig. 10-4B) will confirm the displacement, and is essential for a full evaluation. If a fracture is not seen on a routine AP and lateral view, a view with the femur held in internal rotation helps to visualize the femoral neck and will often reveal a non-displaced fracture. It is also important to evaluate the trabecular pattern of the femoral head and neck; any disruption of the trabecular line is a fracture until proven otherwise.

COMPLICATIONS

The incidence of complications is significant with displaced fractures. Late segmental collapse (avascular necrosis) and non-union each occur in up to 20 percent of cases.

TREATMENT

The patient can be stabilized temporarily with skin traction and bedrest. Undisplaced fractures are pinned *in situ.* Depending on the fracture and the preference of the surgeon, reduction and internal fixation or endoprosthetic replacement are required for displaced fractures.

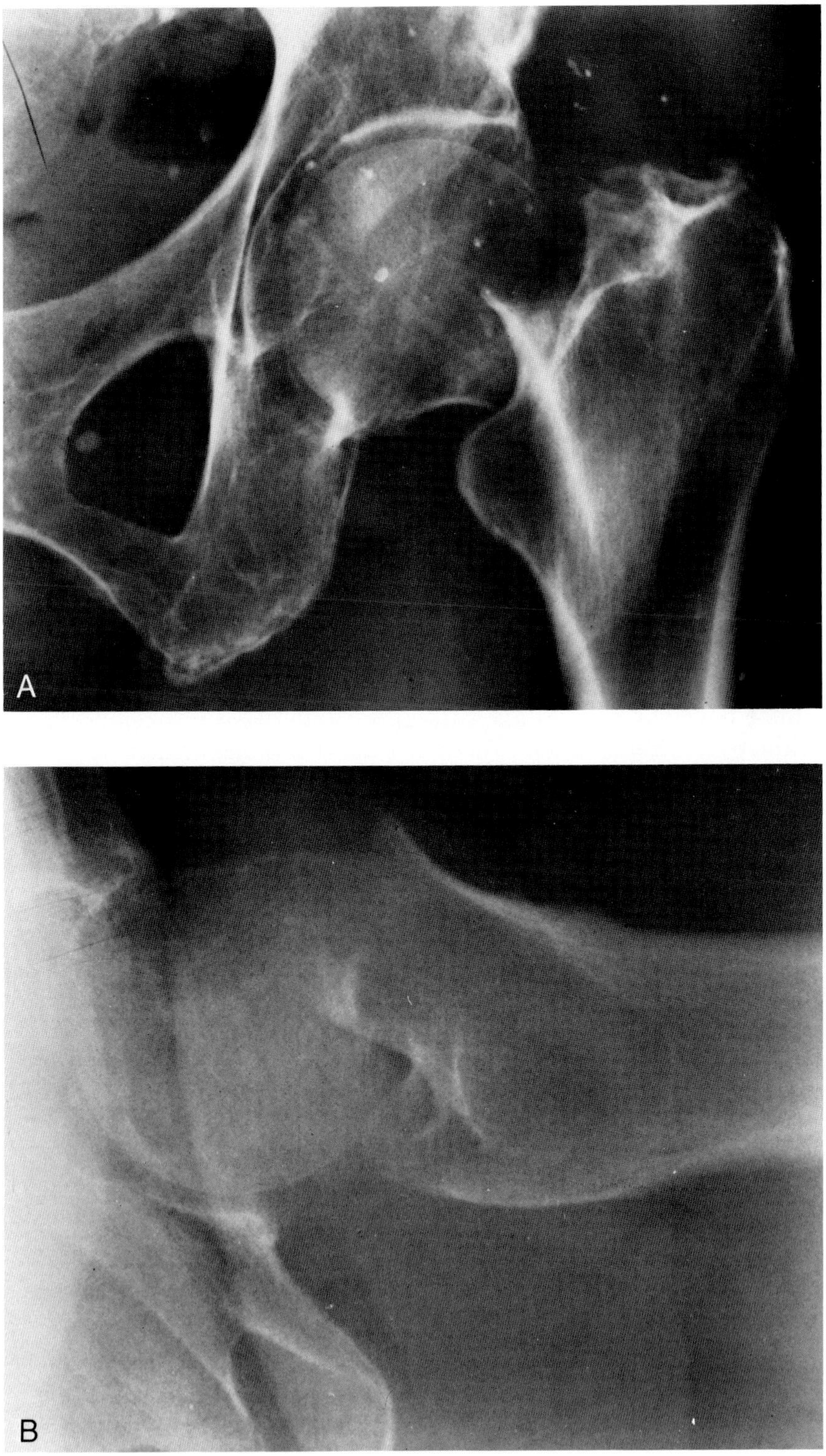

Fig. 10-4. Subcapital fracture. (A) AP view. (B) Lateral view. Note the displacement of the femoral head in both views.

Extracapsular Fractures

The most common extracapsular fracture of the hip is the intertrochanteric fracture. (The two words are often used interchangeably.)

MECHANISM

Similar to neck fracture. Most often a fall in the elderly. High energy trauma in young adults.

CLINICAL PRESENTATION

Displaced fractures present with a shortened and externally rotated leg (Fig. 10-2). The thigh may be swollen from bleeding at the fracture site. The patient resists motion of the injured leg.

ROENTGENOGRAMS

AP and lateral roentgenograms (Figs. 10-5, 10-6). The cross-table lateral film should be obtained, since it helps the surgeon to determine the position and comminution of the fracture. There may be two, three, or four fracture fragments. An AP roentgenogram of the pelvis should also be taken to exclude an associated pelvic fracture.

COMPLICATIONS

Significant blood loss occurs with this fracture and must be replaced. There is a high incidence of associated fractures of the pubic rami. Be careful not to overlook an associated femoral shaft fracture in the multiple trauma patient.

TREATMENT

Initial immobilization with skin traction. Open reduction and internal fixation is the definitive treatment. The method of fixation will depend on the comminution and stability of the fracture.

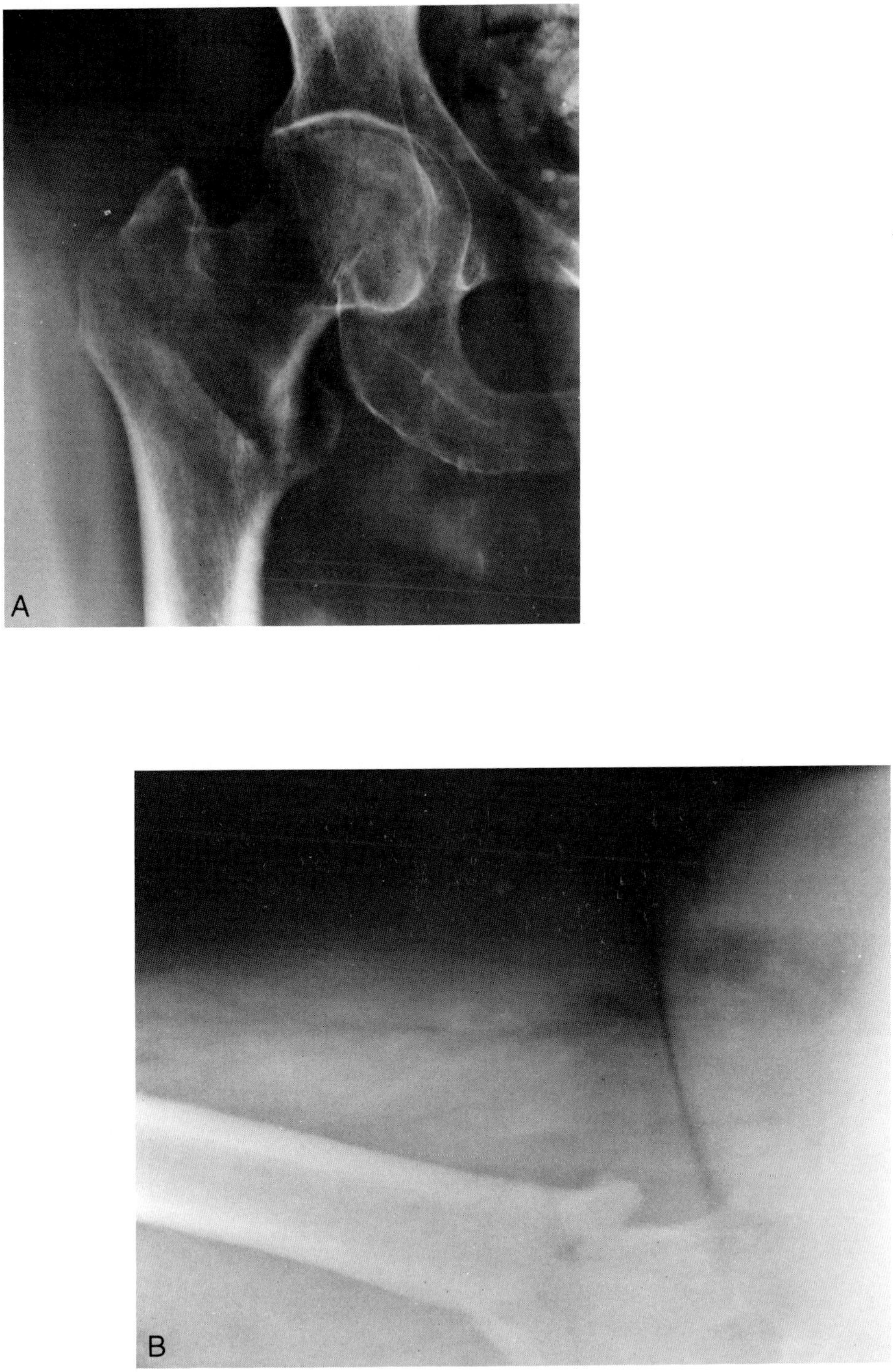

Fig. 10-5. Intertrochanteric fracture (stable). (A) AP view. (B) Lateral view.

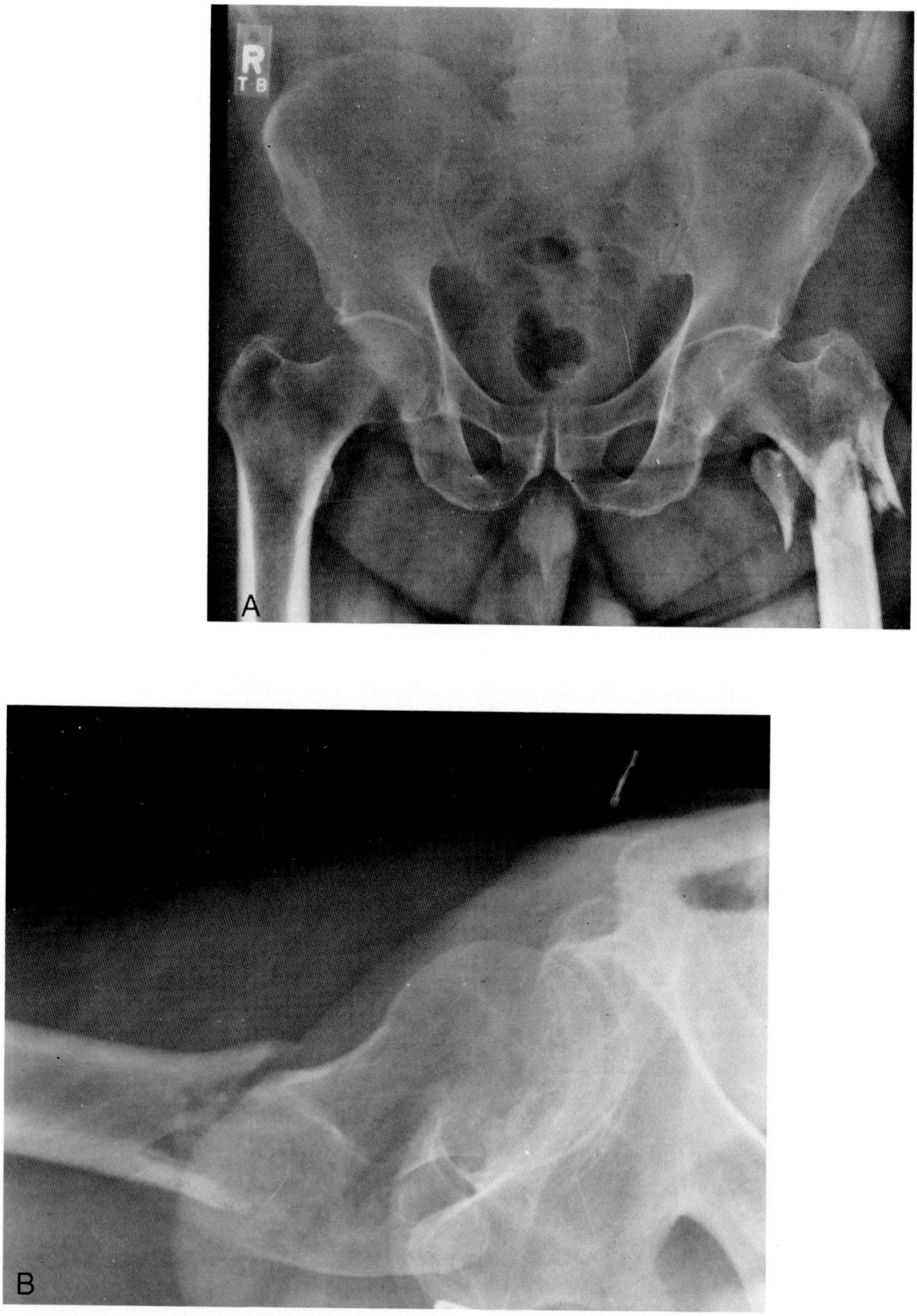

Fig. 10-6. Four-part intertrochanteric fracture. (A) AP view. The four parts include the head and neck, the greater trochanter, the lesser trochanter, and the shaft. (B) Lateral view. This fracture is unstable when reduced because of the medial comminution.

Greater Trochanter Fractures

MECHANISM

These fractures are usually the result of a fall or direct blow to the hip and are often undisplaced.

CLINICAL PRESENTATION

The patient complains of pain in the hip. Ambulation is possible, with difficulty, in some patients. Motion of the hip is uncomfortable, but not extremely painful.

ROENTGENOGRAMS

AP and lateral roentgenograms will reveal the fracture line (Fig. 10-7). It is imperative to exclude the extension of the fracture line through the intertrochanteric area. Tomograms are usually required.

COMPLICATIONS

Misdiagnosis of an intertrochanteric fracture may allow a nondisplaced fracture to displace.

TREATMENT

Symptomatic with partial weight-bearing with crutches as tolerated.

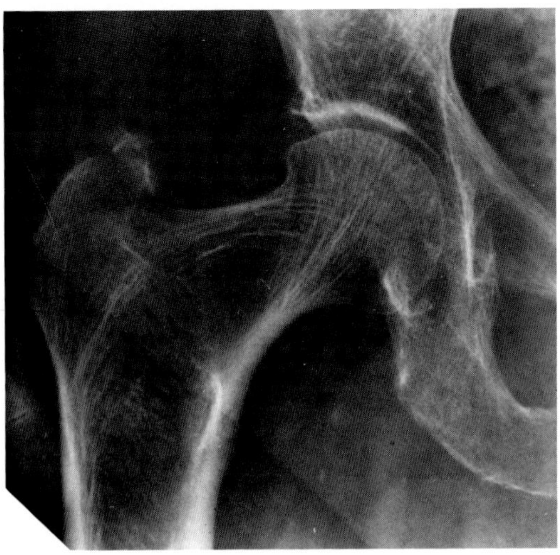

Figure 10-7. Greater trochanter fracture.

Lesser Trochanter Fractures

These fractures are even less common than fractures of the greater trochanter.

MECHANISM

Vigorous physical activity in an adolescent or young adult leads to avulsion of the lesser trochanter.

CLINICAL PRESENTATION

Pain in the groin, especially with abduction or flexion of the hip.

ROENTGENOGRAMS

AP roentgenograms will reveal the fracture (Fig. 10-8). Again, it is essential to determine that no intertrochanteric component exists.

TREATMENT

Symptomatic relief with analgesics, rest, and protected weight-bearing.

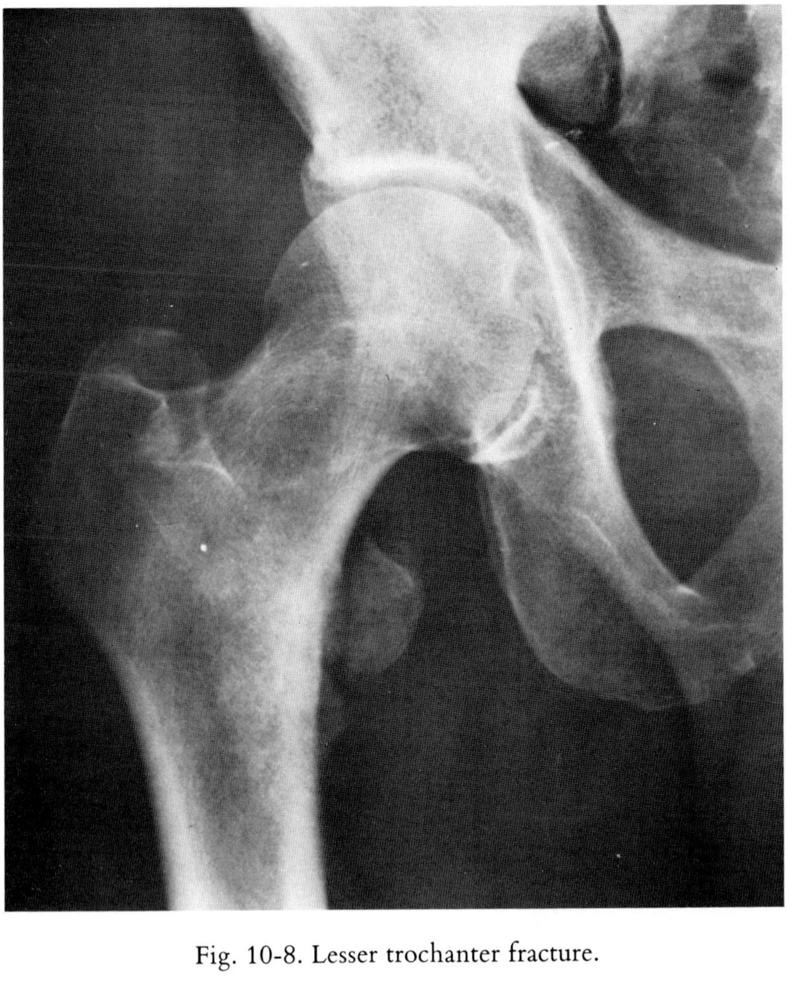

Fig. 10-8. Lesser trochanter fracture.

Subtrochanteric Fractures

Subtrochanteric fractures, by definition, extend below the lesser trochanter. Subtrochanteric fractures may be present as the extension of an intertrochanteric fracture, as an isolated injury, or associated with another femoral fracture.

MECHANISM

Similar to the intertrochanteric fracture.

CLINICAL PRESENTATION

Similar to the intertrochanteric fracture with shortening and external rotation of the leg.

ROENTGENOGRAMS

AP and lateral views reveal the injury. It is important that films of the pelvis and femoral shaft also be obtained.

COMPLICATIONS

Like all femoral and hip fractures, there is significant blood loss from the fracture. Neurovascular injury is rare. Due to the high incidence of deep vein thrombosis, appropriate prophylaxis is indicated for these injuries.

TREATMENT

Open reduction and internal fixation or closed treatment with traction, depending on the surgeon, the fracture, and the patient.

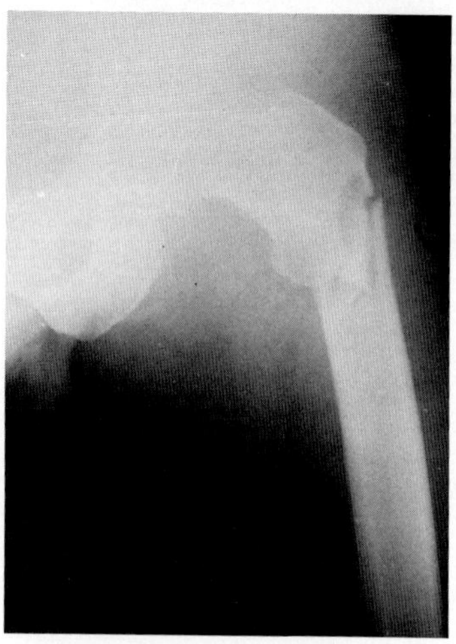

Fig. 10-8A. Subtrochanteric fracture.

HIP DISLOCATIONS

In contrast to hip fractures, dislocations predominate in younger individuals and require significant force. Hip dislocations account for 13 percent of all dislocations. Nerve injury and avascular necrosis are significant problems associated with hip dislocation.

Anterior Dislocations

The anterior dislocation of the hip is less common than posterior.

MECHANISM

Forced abduction of the hip, usually associated with a fall or motor vehicle accident, is the most common etiology.

CLINICAL PRESENTATION

There is little shortening of the affected extremity. The femoral head is palpable anteriorly as a bulge in the groin.

ROENTGENOGRAMS

An AP roentgenogram will reveal the dislocation (Fig. 10-9). A lateral roentgenogram may be obtained to further define the position: anterior, obturator or posterior. The femoral head may appear larger than the contralateral head when the hip is dislocated anteriorly.

COMPLICATIONS

Neurovascular injury may occur, but is less common than in the posterior dislocation.

TREATMENT

Prompt reduction of the dislocation; this usually requires general anesthesia.

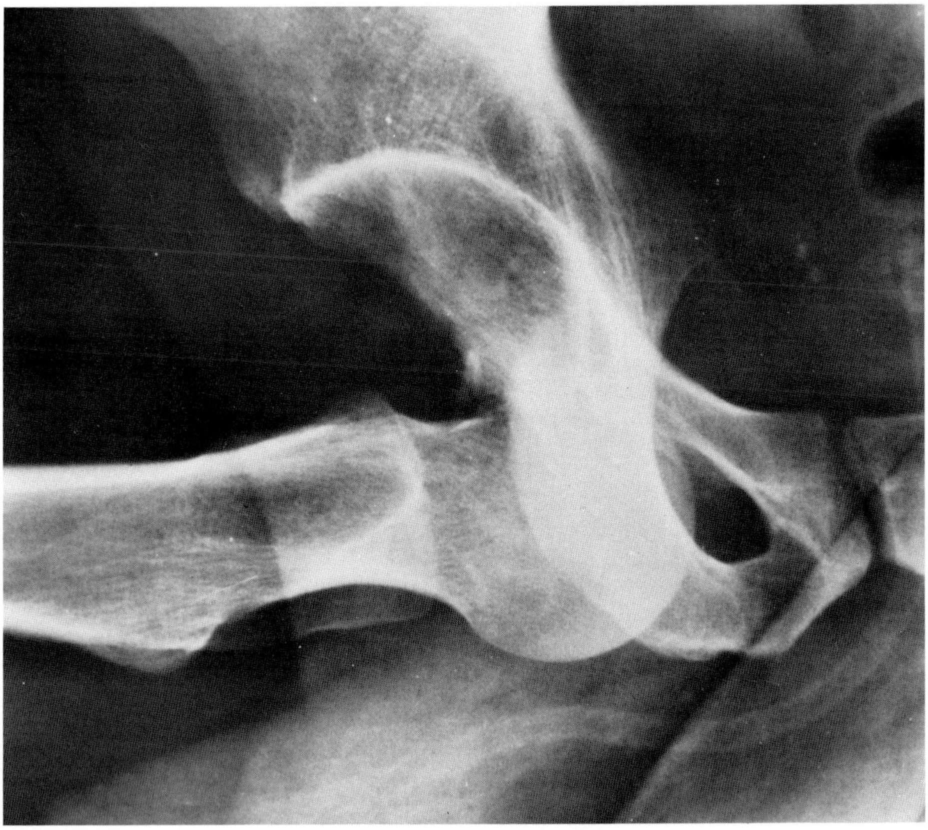

Fig. 10-9. Anterior dislocation of the hip, AP view . The femoral head overlies the pubic ramus, near the obturator fossa.

Posterior Dislocations

MECHANISM

Posterior dislocations of the hip most often results from the flexed knee striking the dashboard in an automobile accident. The greater the flexion of the hip at the time of injury, the less the incidence of associated posterior wall fracture (c.f. Fig. 9-4). Fractures of both the femoral head and acetabulum may occur with posterior dislocation.

CLINICAL PRESENTATION

The patient presents with the leg shortened, abducted, and internally rotated.

ROENTGENOGRAMS

Routine AP view (Fig. 10-10) of the pelvis reveals the dislocation. A 45 degree internal and external oblique view will help determine the extent of the acetabular fracture. The posteriorly dislocated femoral head may appear smaller than the opposite femoral head.

COMPLICATIONS

Sciatic or peroneal nerve injury occurs in 10 to 13 percent of patients. Aseptic necrosis results in 10 to 25 percent of patients. The elapsed time until reduction correlates directly with the incidence of aseptic necrosis. One should be cautious not to miss a hip dislocation when there is a femoral shaft or patellar fracture.

TREATMENT

Prompt reduction of the dislocation; this often requires general anesthesia. Repeated attempts at a closed reduction are contraindicated.
(See the section on *Acetabular Fracture* for the central fracture dislocation.)

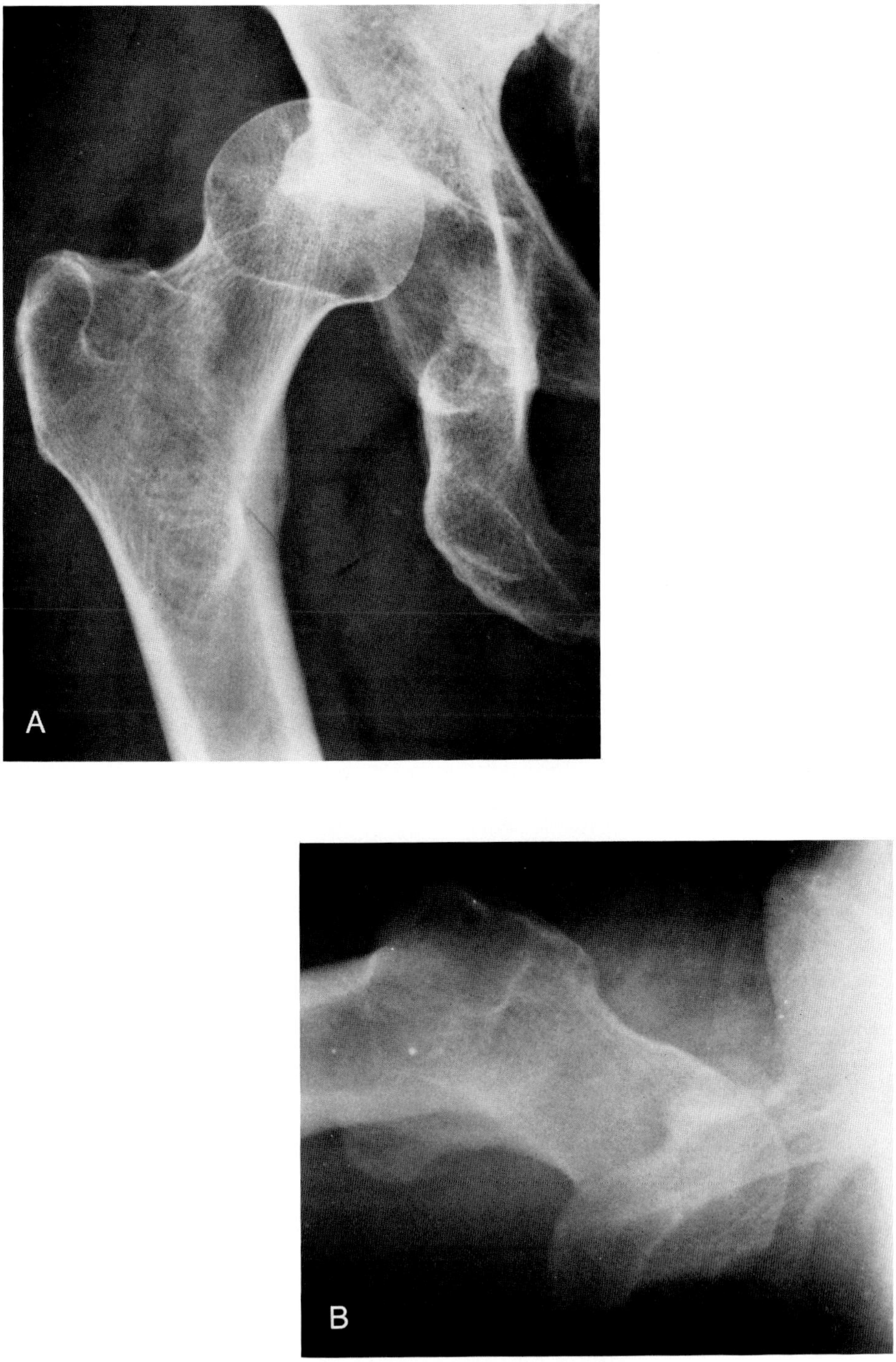

Fig. 10-10. Posterior dislocation of the hip. (A) AP view. The dislocated femoral head may be seen superior and posterior to the acetabulum. (B) Lateral view shows the head to be positioned posterior to the acetabulum and overlying the ischial tuberosity.

Femur Fractures

Fracture of the femur requires significant force. It is most frequently seen in young adults, due to motor vehicle accidents, vigorous athletics, and gunshot wounds. AP (Fig. 10-11A) and lateral views (Fig. 10-11B) should include the hip and knee to ensure that an associated dislocation is not missed.

MECHANISM

Torsional stress produces a spiral fracture. A direct blow will cause a transverse or short oblique fracture. As the forces increase, comminution of the fracture is produced.

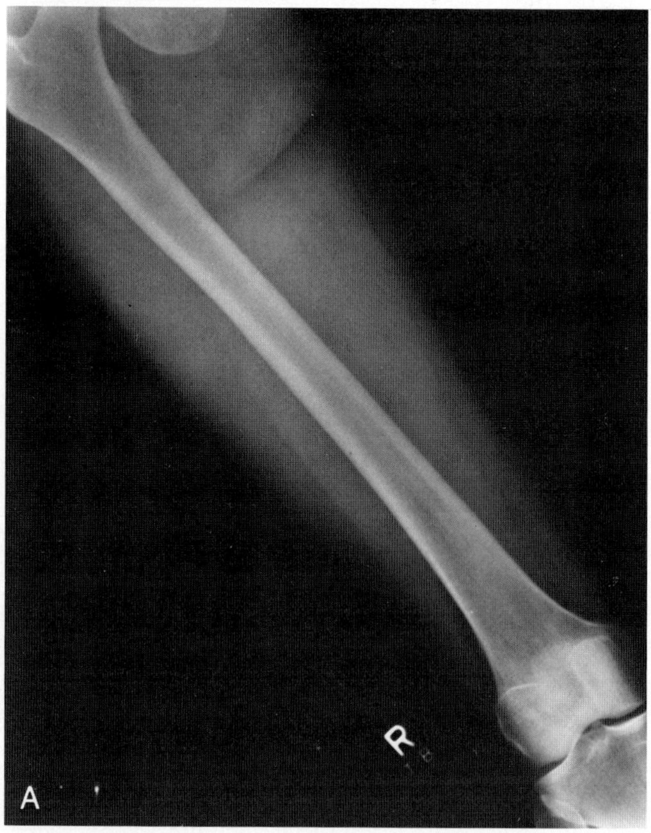

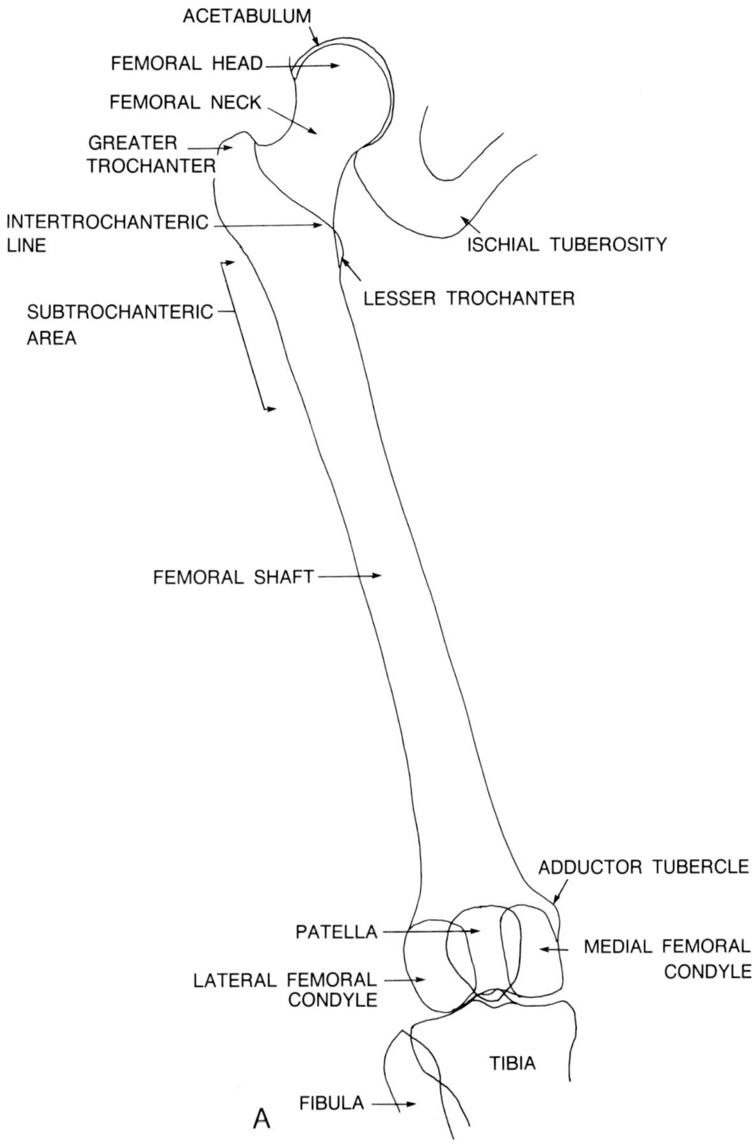

Fig. 10-11. (A) AP view of the femur — normal (Figure continues).

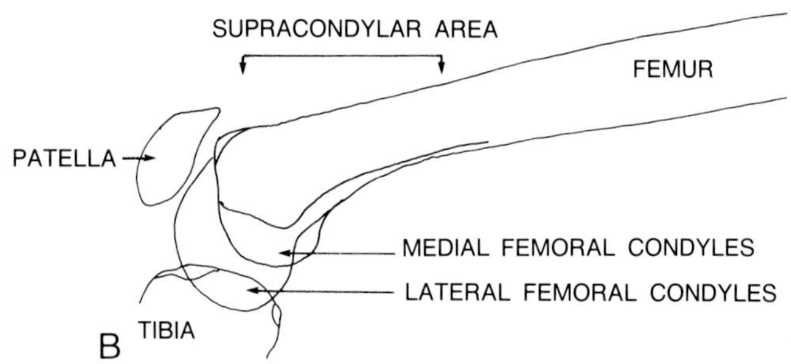

(DISTAL FEMUR)

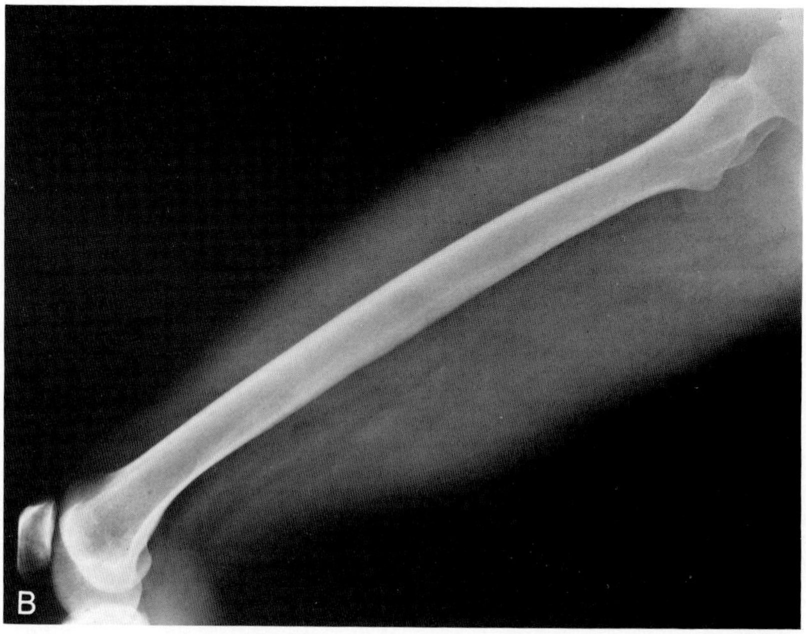

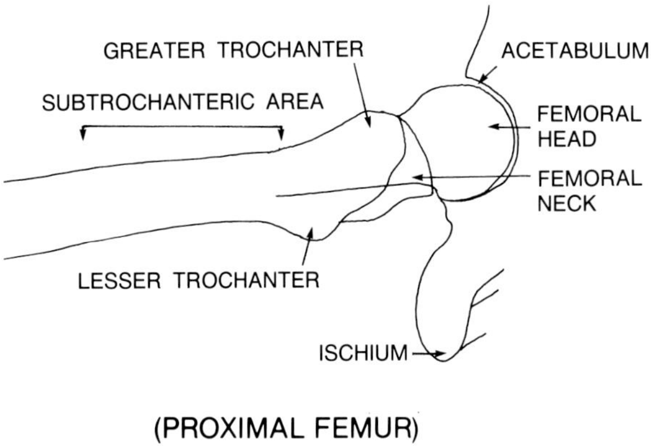

Fig. 10-11 (Continued). (B) Lateral view of the femur — normal.

CLINICAL PRESENTATION

The patient has severe pain, swelling and shortening. The rotation and deformity depend on the site of the fracture and resultant muscle pulls. Hip and knee motion are greatly reduced. Neurovascular injury is rare except in open injuries.

ROENTGENOGRAMS

An AP and lateral view (Fig. 10-12) are adequate for evaluation of the injury. The hip and knee joints must be seen. An AP view of the pelvis should also be obtained to exclude any associated pelvic fractures.

COMPLICATIONS

Hemorrhage in the range of 1 to 2 units of blood occurs from the fracture. Vascular injuries are most common in distal femoral fractures and occur at the adductor hiatus. Deep vein thrombosis is quite common and is increased fivefold in patients over 40. Nerve injury is usually a neuropraxia due to displacement and traction on the nerve. Dislocation of the hip and pelvic fractures should not be overlooked. There is a significant incidence of concomitant closed head injury. Any femoral fracture resulting from minor trauma must be suspected of being pathological.

TREATMENT

Emergency treatment of a femoral fracture requires intravenous resuscitation and blood replacement as needed, and immobilization. Skeletal traction or internal fixation is the definitive treatment.

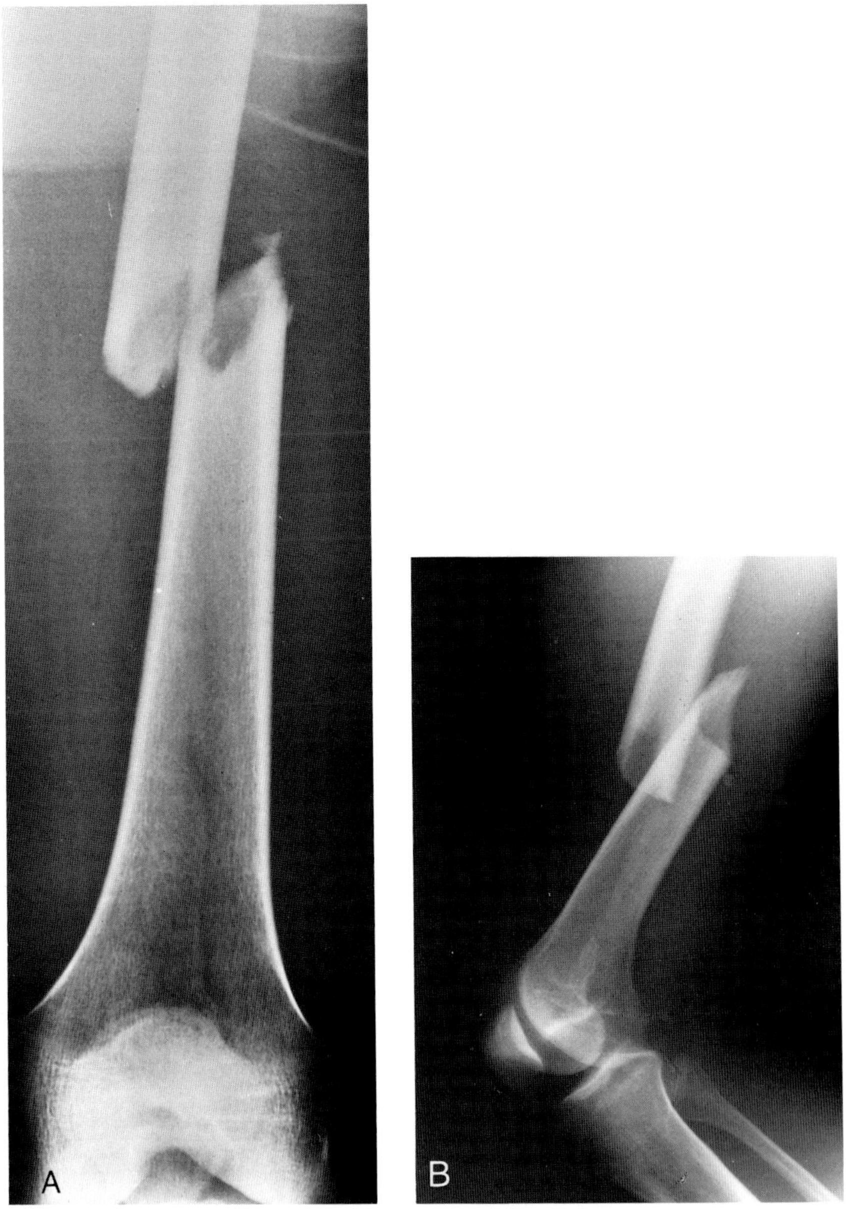

Fig. 10-12. Femoral shaft fracture. (A) AP view. (B) Lateral view.

11 The Knee

Injuries about the knee include fractures of the femoral condyles, patella, and tibial plateaus, as well as injuries to the ligaments and menisci. Routine radiographic examination of the knee consists of the AP view (Fig. 11-1A) and lateral view (Fig. 11-1B). The oblique view (Fig. 11-1C), sunrise view (Fig. 11-1D), and tunnel view (Fig. 11-1E) may also be useful in delineating specific injuries.

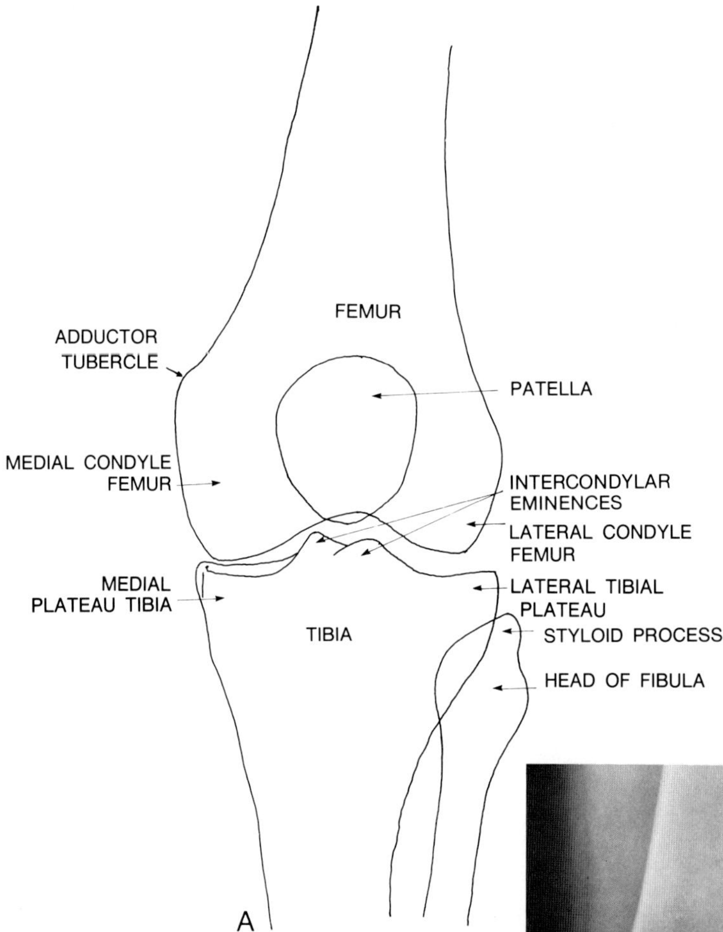

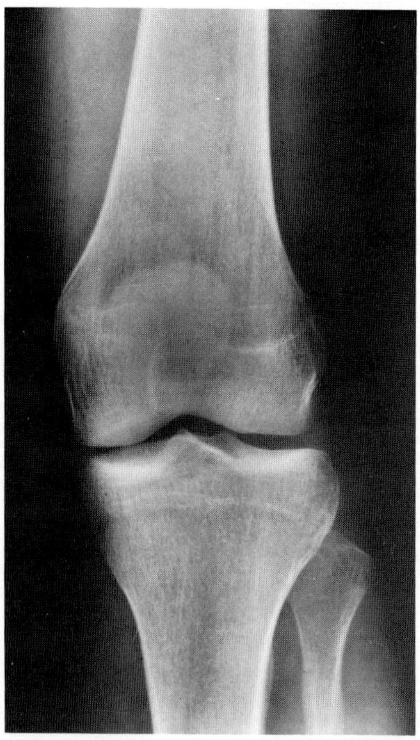

Fig. 11-1. (A) AP view of the knee—normal. (B) Lateral view of knee—normal (Figure continues).

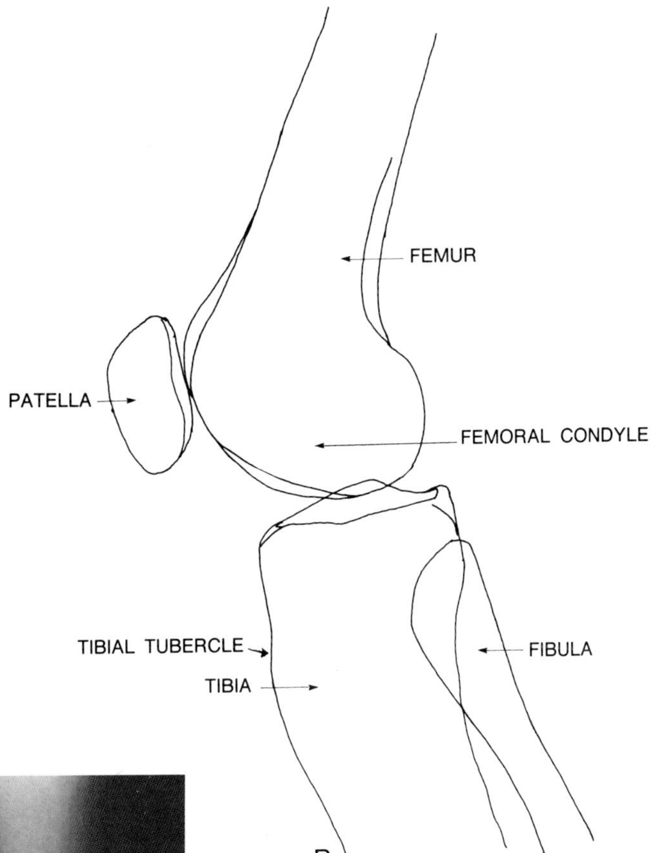
FEMUR
PATELLA
FEMORAL CONDYLE
TIBIAL TUBERCLE
TIBIA
FIBULA

B

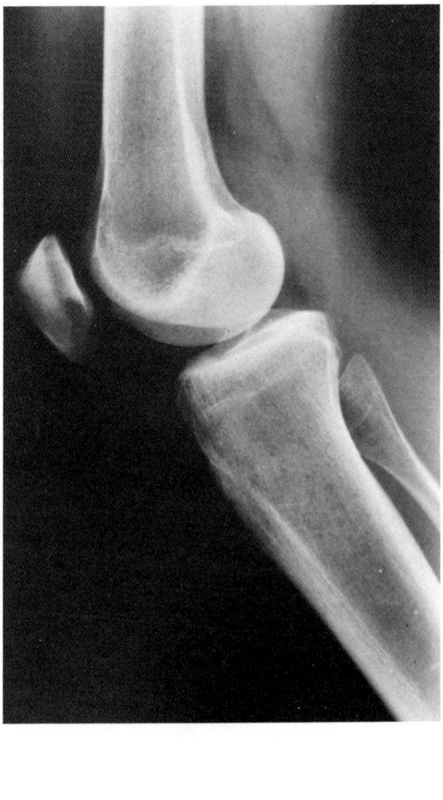

B

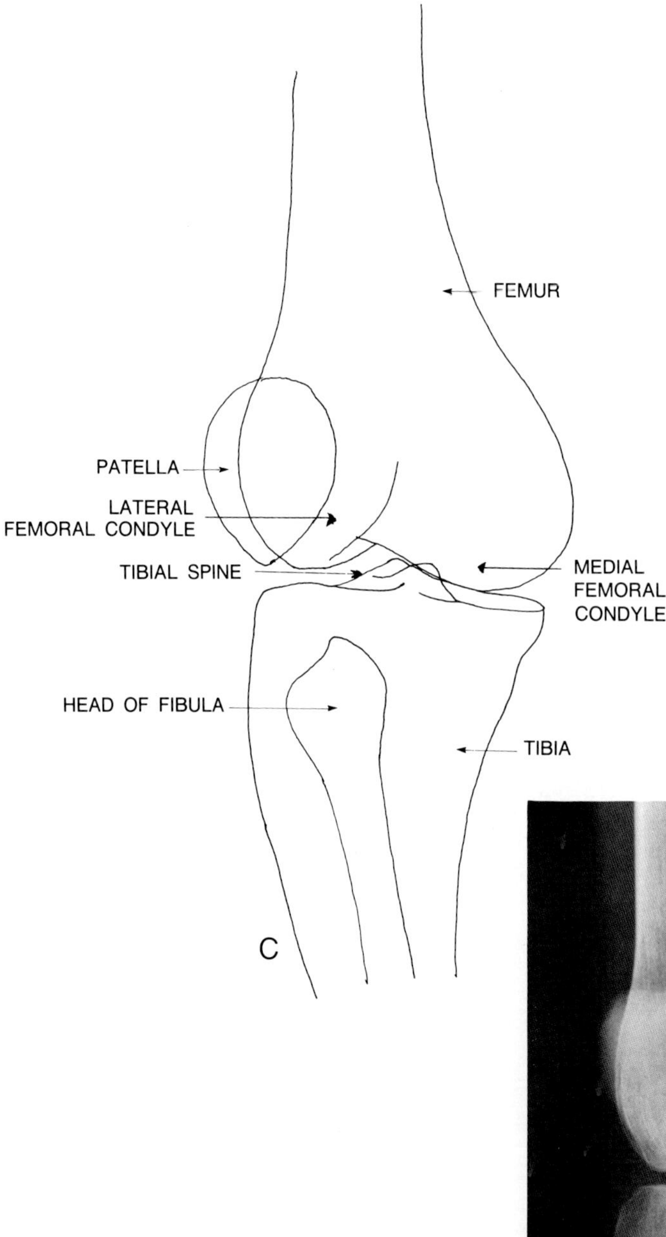

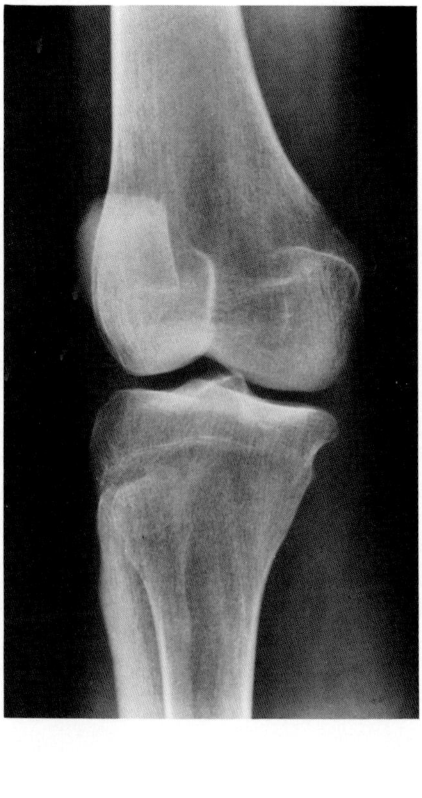

C

Fig. 11-1 (Continued). (C) Oblique view of knee — normal. (D) Sunrise (patellar view) — normal. (E) Intercondylar (tunnel) view of the knee — normal.

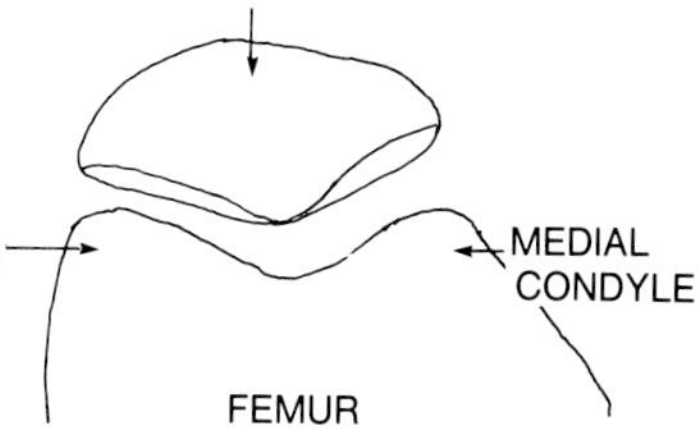

D

PATELLA VIEW

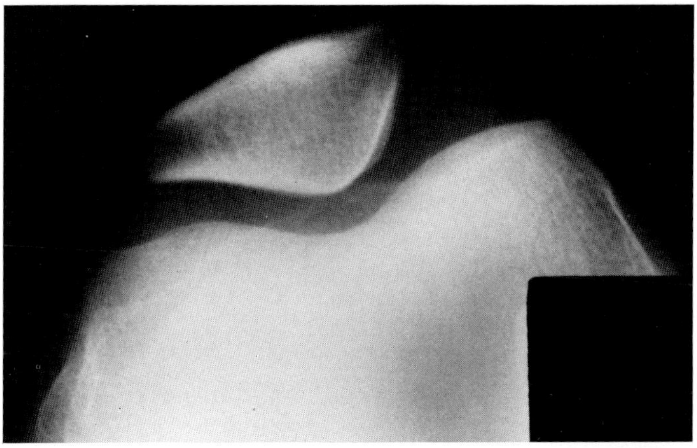

D

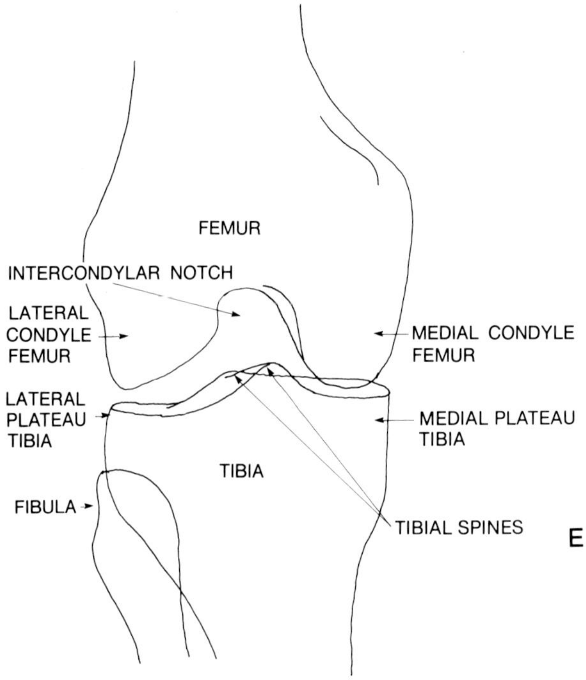

E

INTERCONDYLAR VIEW (TUNNEL)

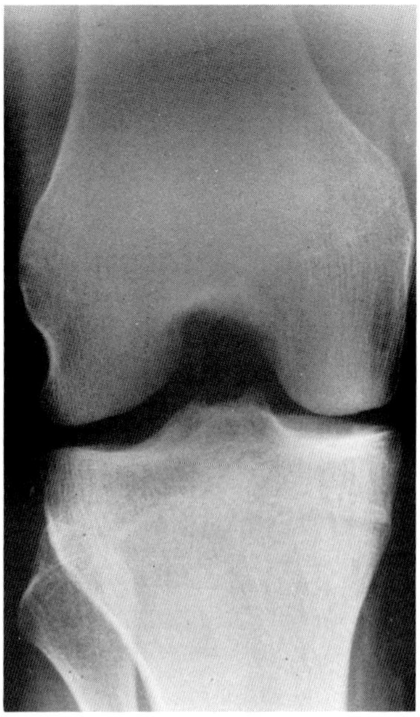

E

Fracture of the Distal Femur

Fractures may involve the condyles or the supracondylar area. They are usually intraarticular.

MECHANISM

Rotary stresses or occasionally a direct blow to the knee. The position of the knee and the direction of the force determine the type and severity of the fracture.

CLINICAL PRESENTATION

The patient presents with knee pain, obvious effusion, and inability to flex or extend the knee. If the joint is aspirated, a bloody effusion is found, which may contain fat globules. Failure to see fat is an unreliable sign.

ROENTGENOGRAMS

AP and lateral roentgenograms (Fig. 11-2) are usually sufficient. If additional information is necessary, obliques and a tunnel view may be obtained.

COMPLICATIONS

Disruption of the congruity of the knee joint. Injury to the popliteal artery.

TREATMENT

Immobilization for undisplaced fractures. Displaced intraarticular fractures require reduction, either by skeletal traction or open reduction and internal fixation.

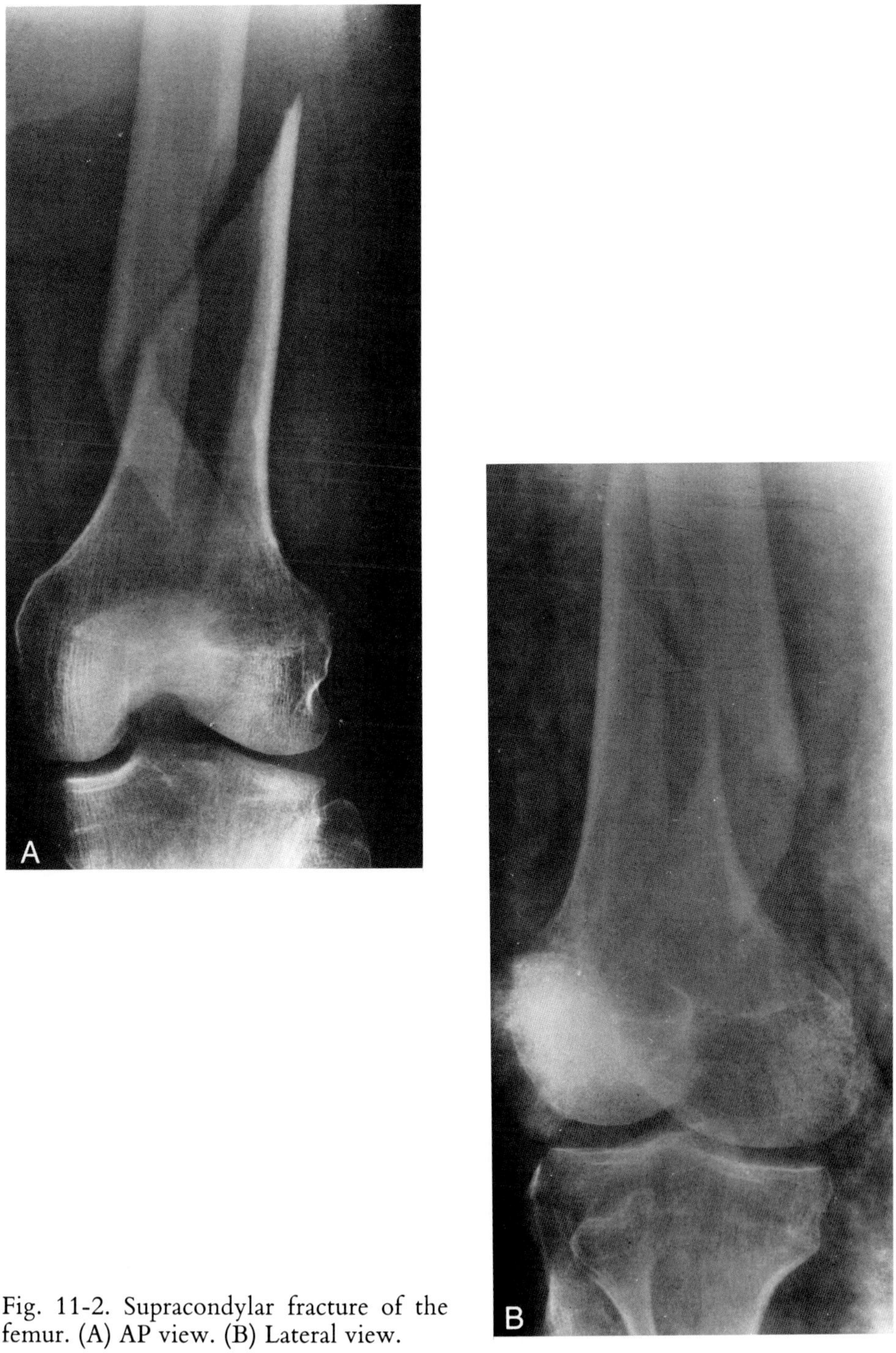

Fig. 11-2. Supracondylar fracture of the femur. (A) AP view. (B) Lateral view.

Patella Fractures

Fracture of the patella accounts for 1 percent of skeletal injuries.

MECHANISM

Direct trauma: a fall on the flexed knee or a direct blow to the patella. Indirect trauma: violent contraction of the quadriceps muscle.

CLINICAL PRESENTATION

Pain and swelling of the knee. There may be a palpable defect in the patella. The patient is unable to extend the knee if the extensor mechanism has been disrupted.

ROENTGENOGRAMS

AP and lateral views of the knee will reveal the fracture (Fig. 11-3). Patellar fractures are considered significantly displaced if the fragments are separated more than 4 mm or if there is an articular step-off of more than 2 mm. A bipartite patella (an unfused, secondary ossification center) may be mistaken for a fracture. The unfused segment is most often at the superlateral pole and is frequently bilateral. A fracture in this area may be assumed to be a bipartite patella if it is bilateral.

COMPLICATIONS

Neurovascular injuries are rare but associated injuries to the hip, pelvis, and femur should be ruled out. One must consider the diagnosis of quadriceps rupture in the patient with negative roentgenograms who is unable to extend the knee. The defect in the quadriceps is usually palpable.

TREATMENT

Displaced fractures require open reduction and internal fixation. Undisplaced fractures may be treated with immobilization.

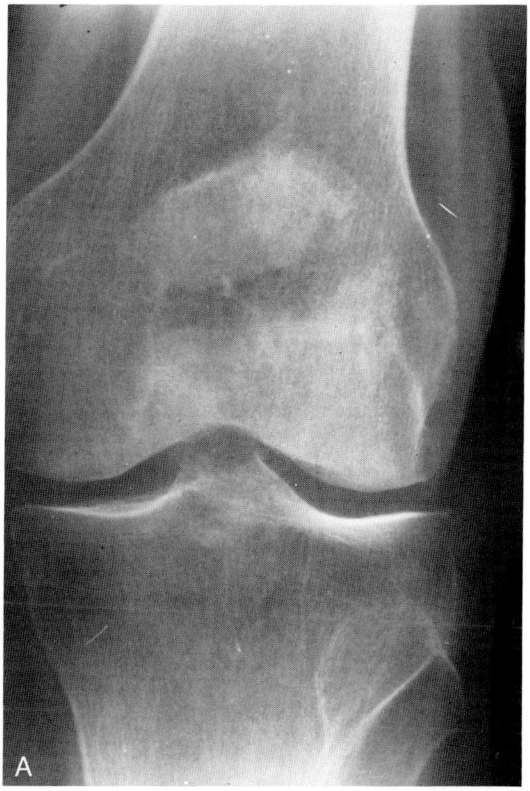

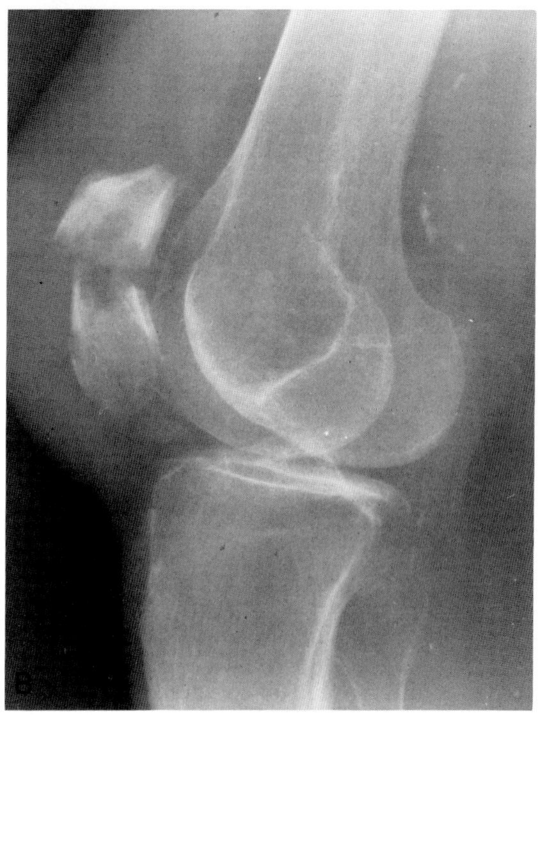

Fig. 11-3. Patellar fracture. (A) AP view. (B) Lateral view. Patellar fractures displace due to the pull of the quadriceps muscle.

Tibial Plateau Fractures

MECHANISM

The combination of compression by the femur with varus or valgus stress on the lateral or medial plateau, as when the knee is struck from the side. (Hence the name "bumper fracture.") Also axial loading, as in a fall from a height.

CLINICAL PRESENTATION

The patient presents with a painful, swollen knee and tenderness over the fractured plateau. Medial-lateral instability is due to the compression of the fracture and/or frequently associated ligamentous injuries.

ROENTGENOGRAMS

AP and lateral views (Fig. 11-4) usually reveal the fracture. Oblique roentgenograms or a film taken at 105 degrees to the shaft of the tibia (tibial plateau view) may add more detail. Stress roentgenograms should be performed only by the orthopaedic surgeon. Tomograms may also be necessary.

COMPLICATIONS

Associated injuries include the meniscus and the collateral ligaments. Injury to the peroneal nerve is not uncommon. Anterior or posterior compartment syndrome may occur with severe injuries. The most common combination of injuries is the lateral tibial plateau fracture, lateral meniscus tear, and medial collateral ligament injury.

TREATMENT

A posterior splint or knee immobilizer is satisfactory emergency treatment. If the joint is extremely tense, aspiration of the effusion (hemarthrosis) may be indicated. Minimially displaced fractures are treated by early motion. Significantly displaced fractures (greater than 5 mm depression of the plateau) require open reduction.

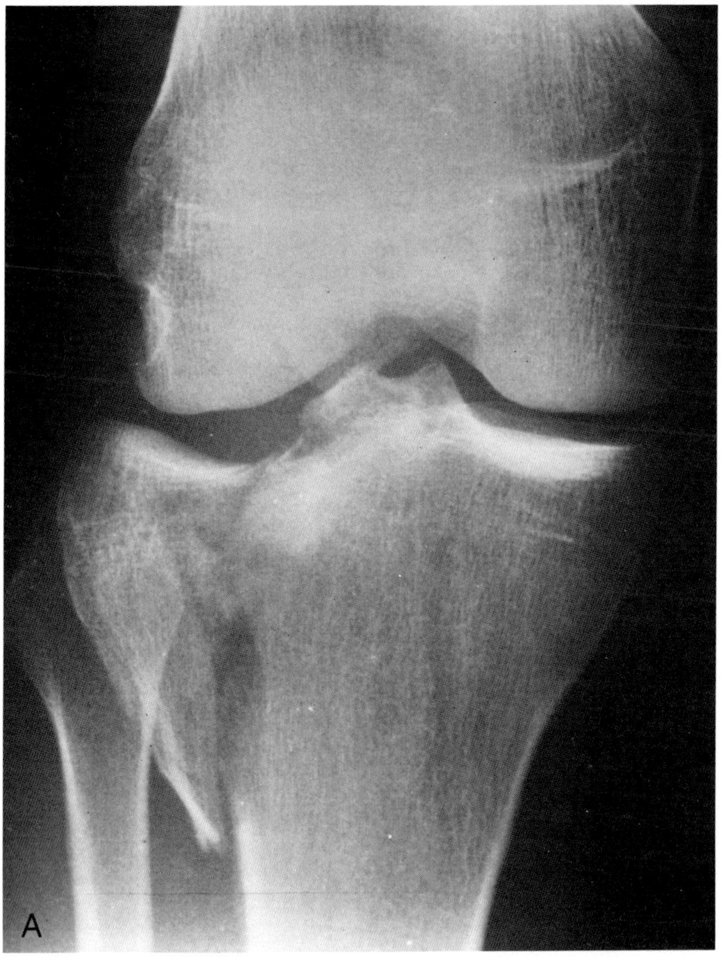

Fig. 11-4. Tibial plateau fracture. (A) AP view of displaced tibial plateau. (Figure continues.)

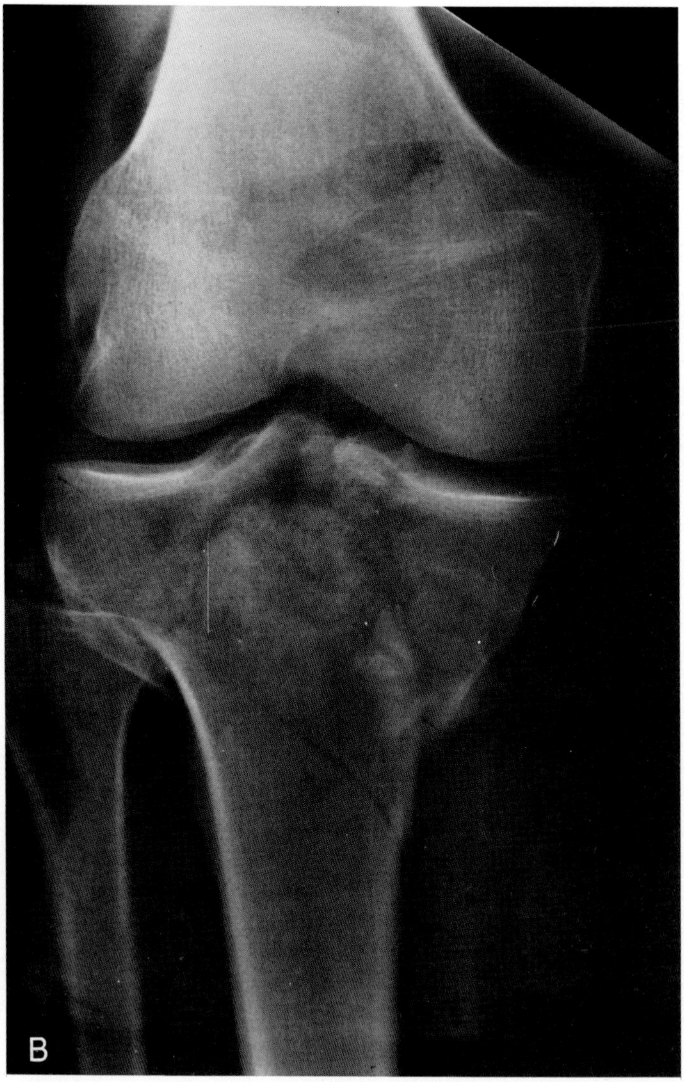

Fig. 11-4(B) (Figure continues).

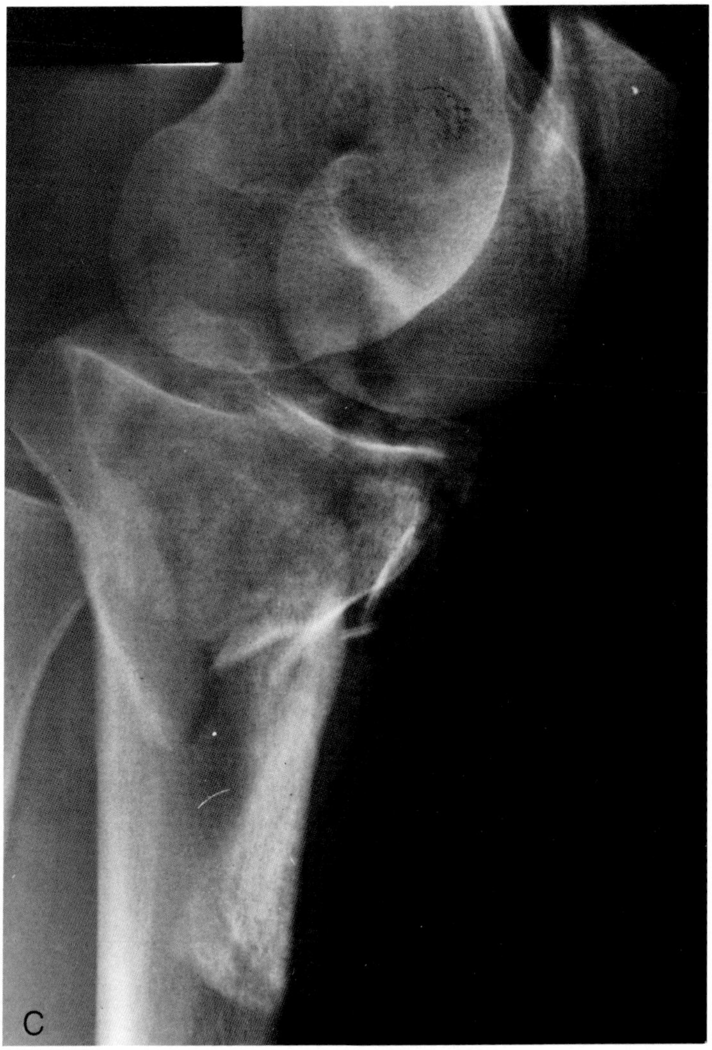

Fig. 11-4 (Continued). Tibial plateau fracture. (B) AP of a complex bicondylar fracture. (C) Lateral of the complex bicondylar fracture.

Knee Dislocation

This rare injury is an orthopaedic emergency.

MECHANISM

High energy trauma with violent abduction and medial rotation of the thigh on the flexed leg. Automobile accidents are the most common cause.

CLINICAL PRESENTATION

The patient presents with a grossly deformed leg. He may be unable to dorsiflex the foot. Distal pulses may be absent, or there may be obvious vascular insufficiency.

ROENTGENOGRAMS

AP and lateral roentgenograms (Fig. 11-5) should be obtained as quickly as possible. If absent pulses do not promptly return after reduction of the knee, an arteriogram should be performed immediately.

COMPLICATIONS

The incidence of vascular injury is 25 to 35 percent. Peroneal nerve injury occurs with a similar incidence. The importance of evaluating these two limb-threatening complications cannot be overemphasized.

TREATMENT

Reduction should be accomplished as quickly as possible, especially in the face of neurovascular compromise. Postreduction evaluation of neurovascular status is essential.

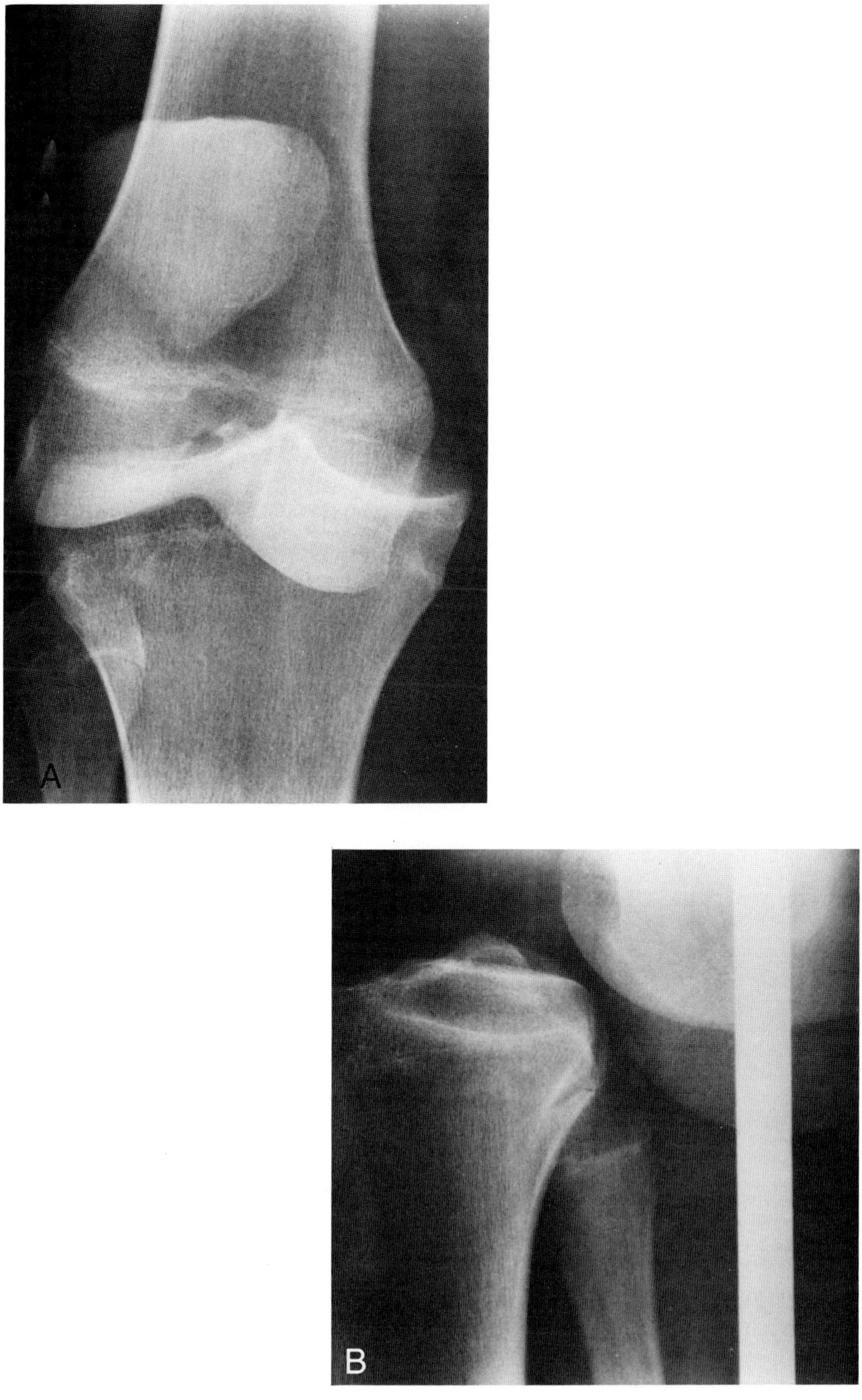

Fig. 11-5. Anterior dislocation of the knee. (A) AP view. (B) Lateral view. This is an orthopaedic emergency, requiring immediate reduction. It carries a high incidence of neurovascular injury.

Patellar Dislocation

MECHANISM

Dislocation of the patella may be caused by violent contraction of the quadriceps or a blow to the patella when the knee is flexed. The patella generally dislocates laterally. Recurrent dislocation is common.

CLINICAL PRESENTATION

The patient may present with a history of previous dislocation. The dislocated patella will often reduce spontaneously. Once the patella is reduced, the patient may have only a swollen knee with tenderness over the medial aspect. The Fairbanks test (apprehension test) is uniformly positive and will help differentiate a meniscal tear and a reduced patellar dislocation. If the patella is not reduced, there will be a prominent lateral femoral condyle. Reduction can generally be achieved by gentle, steady pressure from the lateral side.

ROENTGENOGRAMS

AP, lateral, and sunrise views (Fig. 11-6) should be obtained. Because of the high incidence of spontaneous reduction, the dislocation often cannot be demonstrated radiographically. Post-reduction films are necessary both to confirm the reduction and to identify osteochondral fractures (Fig. 11-7).

COMPLICATIONS

Osteochondral fracture of the patella.

TREATMENT

Reduction of the dislocation by firm pressure on the lateral border of the patella.

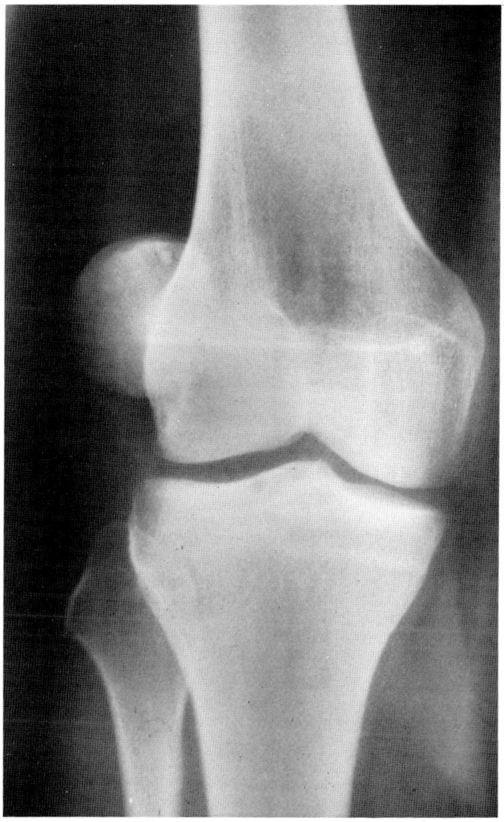

Fig. 11-6. Patellar dislocation. The AP view demonstrates the patella to be dislocated laterally.

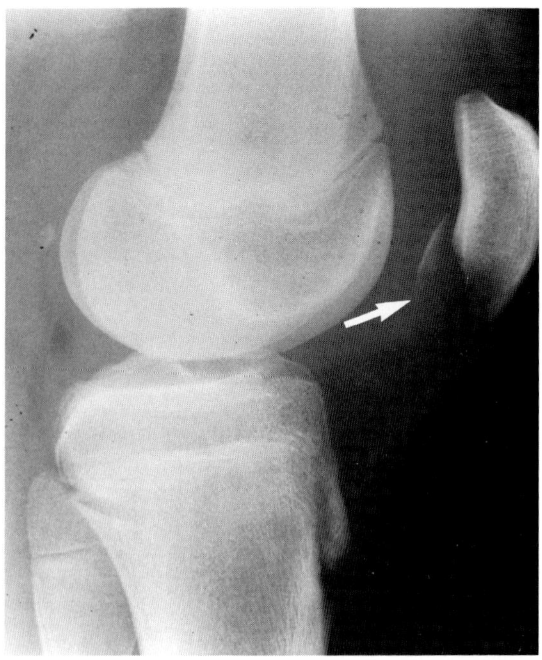

Fig. 11-7. Osteochondral fracture following patellar dislocation. Arrow indicates fracture fragment.

SOFT TISSUE INJURY ABOUT THE KNEE

Injuries to the menisci, collateral, and cruciate ligaments are common. They are often sustained during sports. Both isolated lesions and combined injuries may occur.

Meniscal Injury

Meniscal tear is the most common soft tissue injury to the knee. The medial is more commonly injured than the lateral, at a ratio of 5 : 1.

MECHANISM

Rotation or sudden forceful flexion or extension of the thigh on the fixed leg.

CLINICAL PRESENTATION

Effusion is usually present. "Locking" or inability to fully extend the knee strongly suggests a meniscal injury. Tenderness can be elicited at the joint line on the involved side.

ROENTGENOGRAMS

AP and lateral roentgenograms reveal a joint effusion, but are otherwise negative.

COMPLICATIONS

Associated cruciate and/or collateral ligament injuries should not be overlooked.

TREATMENT

A knee immobilizer is sufficient initial treatment.

Collateral Ligament Injuries

The medial collateral ligament is injured more commonly than the lateral.

MECHANISM

The medial collateral ligament may be injured by a blow from the lateral side, causing a valgus strain on the knee. The less common lateral collateral ligament injury occurs with a varus stress. When combined with a rotatory injury, damage to the cruciate ligament and meniscus can occur. Depending upon the severity of the force and the position of the knee, the patient may suffer a strain, mild stretching, or a frank tear of the ligament.

CLINICAL PRESENTATION

Physical examination will reveal tenderness along the ligament. Instability may be present. Surprisingly, the patient may be able to walk, or have even continued the sports activity after the injury.

ROENTGENOGRAMS

Roentgenograms are usually normal. Rarely one may see a small avulsion at the origin or insertion of the collateral ligament into the bone.

COMPLICATIONS

Misdiagnosis of associated injuries.

TREATMENT

A knee immobilizer will suffice until follow-up or consultation in the emergency room is obtained. Early orthopaedic follow-up is necessary to determine if immobilization or surgery is required.

Cruciate Ligament Injuries

Because a portion of both cruciate ligaments is taut in all degrees of knee flexion, they are susceptible to injury. The anterior cruciate ligament is injured more often than the posterior.

MECHANISM

Anterior cruciate ligament injury is generally produced by a combination of internal rotation and extension. Posterior cruciate ligament injury results from forceful posterior displacement of the proximal tibia with the knee in flexion.

CLINICAL PRESENTATION

An audible "pop" is common. The patient is usually unable to continue further activity. A large effusion is present. Pain cannot be localized and is felt deep within the knee.

ROENTGENOGRAMS

AP and lateral roentgenograms are usually normal. Occasionally an avulsion fracture of the tibial spine at the insertion of the ligament can occur. Care should be taken not to miss an osteochondral fracture, which can produce similar symptoms.

COMPLICATIONS

An anterior cruciate injury is seen more often in combination with other injuries than as an isolated entity. The classic "triad" consists of an anterior cruciate ligament tear, a medial collateral ligament tear, and a medial meniscal tear. These injuries usually require surgery.

TREATMENT

Immobilization of the knee will suffice as a temporary measure. Early evaluation by the orthopaedist is necessary to determine if acute repair is necessary.

12 The Tibia and Fibula

The tibia is the most common long bone to be fractured. Because of its subcutaneous location, fractures of the tibia are frequently open, requiring emergency debridement, as well as immobilization.

MECHANISM

Torsional forces produce spiral or oblique fractures. Direct high energy violence will produce transverse and/or comminuted fractures. A direct blow produces a transverse or comminuted fracture. Indirect trauma with rotation produces a spiral or an oblique fracture.

CLINICAL PRESENTATION

The classical signs of pain, swelling, angular deformity, gross motion, and crepitus. The evaluation of the neurovascular status is essential. Anterior compartment syndrome and neural injury are significant risks.

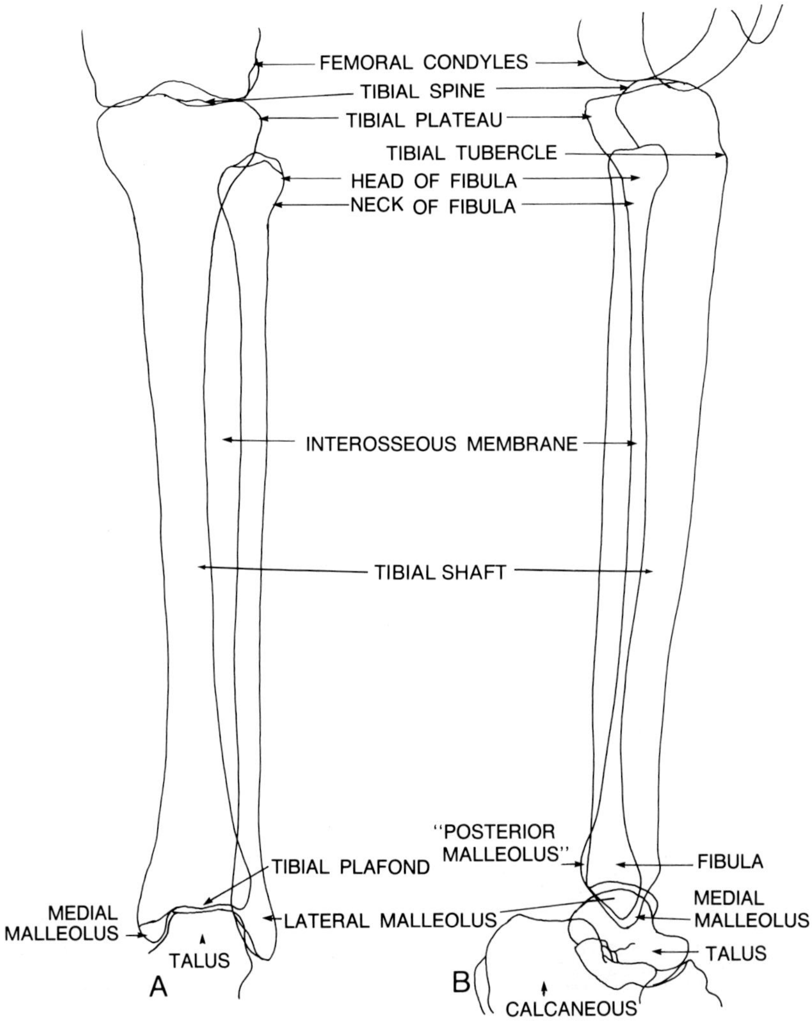
FEMORAL CONDYLES
TIBIAL SPINE
TIBIAL PLATEAU
TIBIAL TUBERCLE
HEAD OF FIBULA
NECK OF FIBULA
INTEROSSEOUS MEMBRANE
TIBIAL SHAFT
"POSTERIOR MALLEOLUS"
TIBIAL PLAFOND
FIBULA
MEDIAL MALLEOLUS
LATERAL MALLEOLUS
MEDIAL MALLEOLUS
TALUS
TALUS
A
B
CALCANEOUS

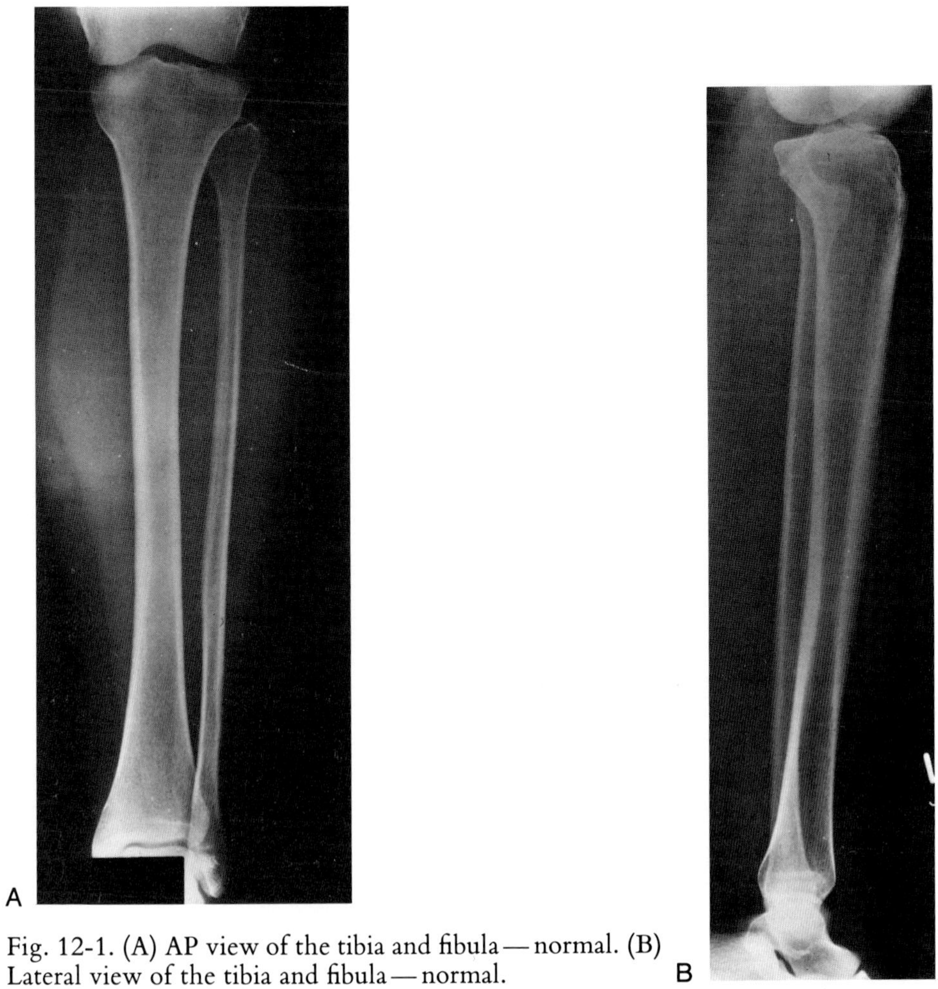

Fig. 12-1. (A) AP view of the tibia and fibula — normal. (B) Lateral view of the tibia and fibula — normal.

ROENTGENOGRAMS

AP and lateral views (Figs. 12-2, 12-3) should include the knee and ankle. Extension of the fracture into the joint with attendant articular disruption must be evaluated and/or excluded. The initial roentgenograms are often the most important films because they reveal the initial displacement of the fracture.

COMPLICATIONS

Neurovascular injuries are not uncommon. A high percentage of tibial fractures are open, carrying the obvious risk of infection. Anterior compartment syndrome may occur in any patient with a tibial fracture, and is more common in closed injuries. Circular casts must be applied with caution and are usually best split to the skin. Failure to anticipate and treat swelling can lead to unnecessary loss of function or even loss of the limb.

TREATMENT

Initial immobilization in a long-leg splint, until seen by the orthopaedist. The vast majority of these patients require admission to the hospital for frequent neurovascular observation. Open fractures require emergency debridement in the operating room.

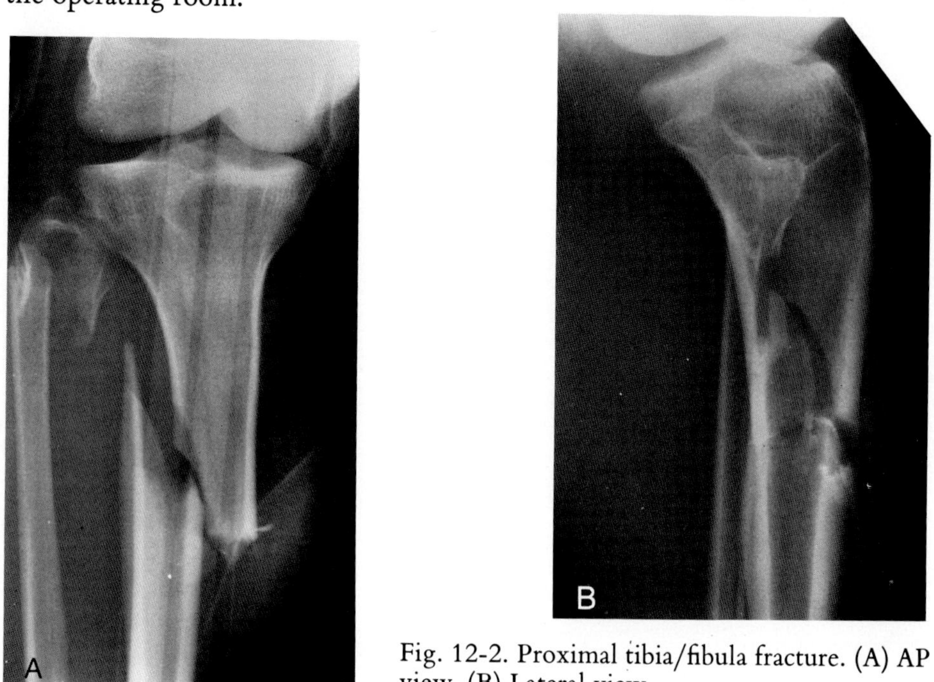

Fig. 12-2. Proximal tibia/fibula fracture. (A) AP view. (B) Lateral view.

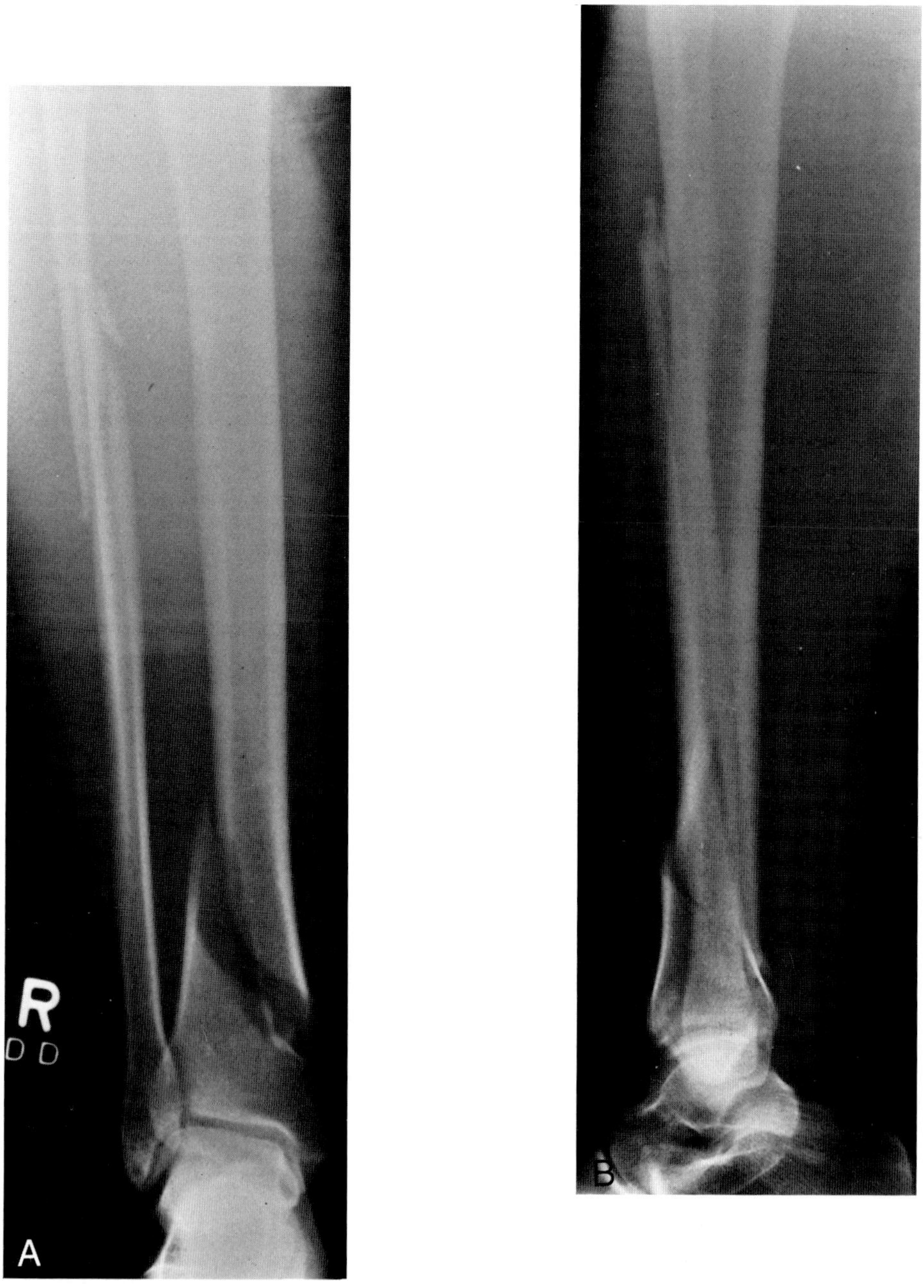

Fig. 12-3. Distal tibia/fibula fracture. (A) AP view. (B) Lateral view. If displacement of the tibia exists, there must be either a fracture of the fibula or dislocation of the fibula at either the knee or ankle joint.

13 The Ankle

MECHANISM

The most common mechanism of ankle injury is supination, adduction, and internal rotation; the patient reports "twisting the ankle." The direction and degree of force applied determine both the pattern of the fracture and its severity. Minor forces cause sprains or undisplaced fractures; larger forces create major disruptions of the ankle anatomy.

CLINICAL PRESENTATION

Localized pain, swelling, and ecchymosis are present. Sprains and undisplaced fractures are merely painful. Displaced fractures present with deformity and are often massively swollen. Like the pelvis, the ankle is a ring; it must be broken in two places for significant displacement to occur. Careful search must therefore be made for occult "second side injury" in the patient with obvious injury to a single malleolus (e.g., *deltoid ligament injury* with fracture of the lateral malleolus or *proximal fibular fracture* with "isolated" injury to the deltoid ligament or medial malleolus.

ROENTGENOGRAMS

AP, lateral, and mortise views (15 – 20° of internal rotation) should be obtained (Fig. 13-1). The width of the joint space should be constant around the entire ankle mortise (Fig. 13-2).

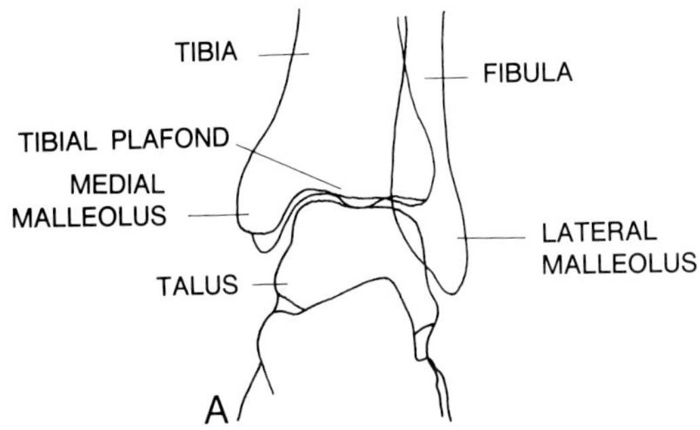

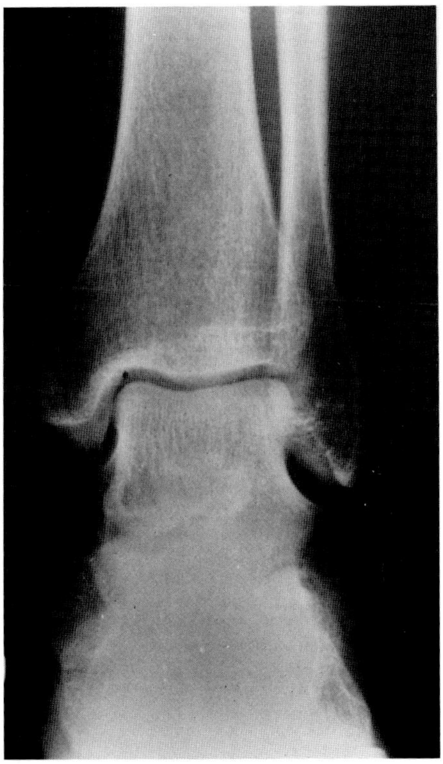

A

Fig. 13-1. (A) AP view of the ankle—normal. (B) Lateral view of the ankle—normal (Figure continues).

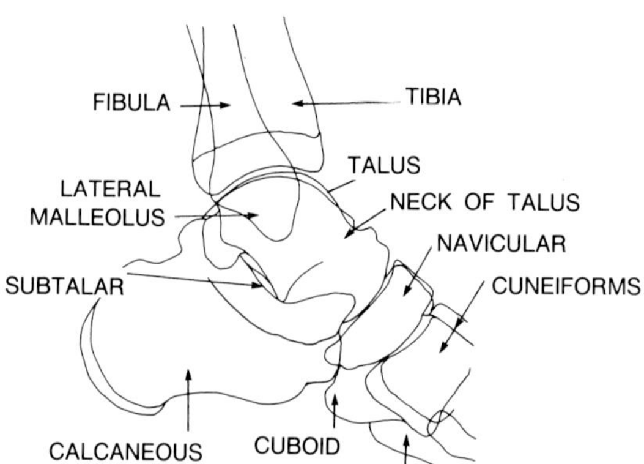

B

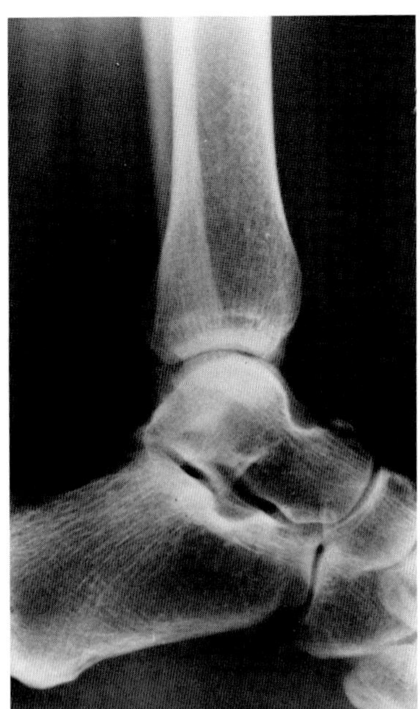

B

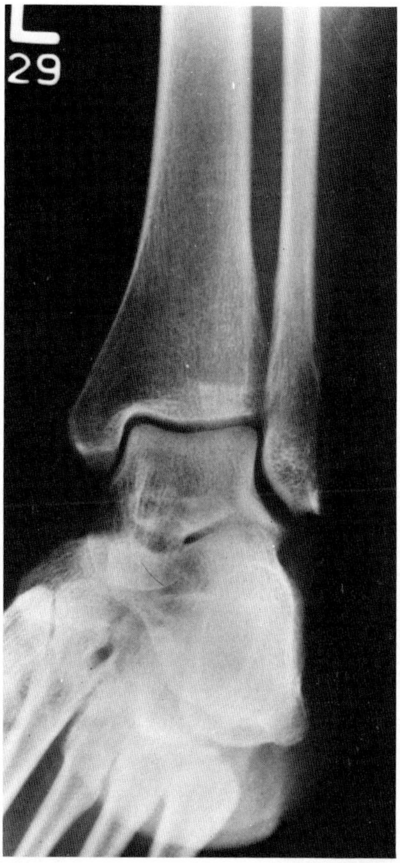

C

Fig. 13-1 (Continued). (C) Mortise (15° internal rotation) view of the ankle—normal.

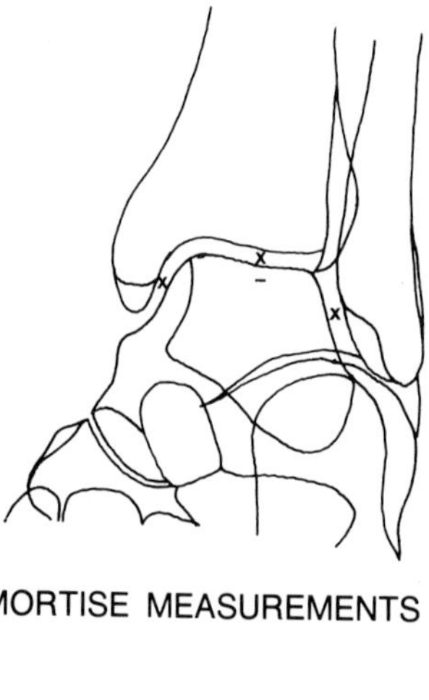

MORTISE MEASUREMENTS X

Fig. 13-2. Mortise view of the ankle. The width of the joint space should remain constant around the talus.

Ankle Sprain

Sprains generally involve injury to the anterior talofibular ligament.

MECHANISM

Inversion and supination of the foot.

CLINICAL PRESENTATION

Pain is localized to the anterolateral aspect of the ankle. If the patient complains of medial pain with a negative roentgenogram, a deltoid ligament injury must be suspected.

ROENTGENOGRAMS

Soft tissue swelling only. The montise is intact and the joint space is symmetrical.

COMPLICATIONS

Failure to diagnose an unstable injury.

TREATMENT

Treatment may vary. Crutches, Ace wrap and early mobilization, protection by strapping or splints, and short leg walking plaster are all satisfactory.

Lateral Malleolar Fracture

Oblique fracture of the lateral malleolus is the most common ankle fracture.

MECHANISM

Supination of the foot.

CLINICAL PRESENTATION

Pain and swelling over the lateral aspect of the ankle. It is imperative to check for medial tenderness, since it may be the only clinical indication of a deltoid ligament injury.

ROENTGENOGRAMS

AP, lateral, and mortise films (Fig. 13-3) should be obtained. A space of greater than 4 mm between the medial malleolus and the talus on the mortise view is suggestive of a deltoid ligament tear (Fig. 13-4). The presence of a deltoid ligament tear with the fibular fracture changes a stable injury to an unstable one and changes the treatment regimen.

COMPLICATIONS

Failure to diagnose an associated deltoid ligament injury.

TREATMENT

The undisplaced lateral malleolar fracture can be treated with a short-leg walking cast. Significant displacement indicates a second break in the "ring" of the ankle, and requires reduction and immobilization in long leg plaster.

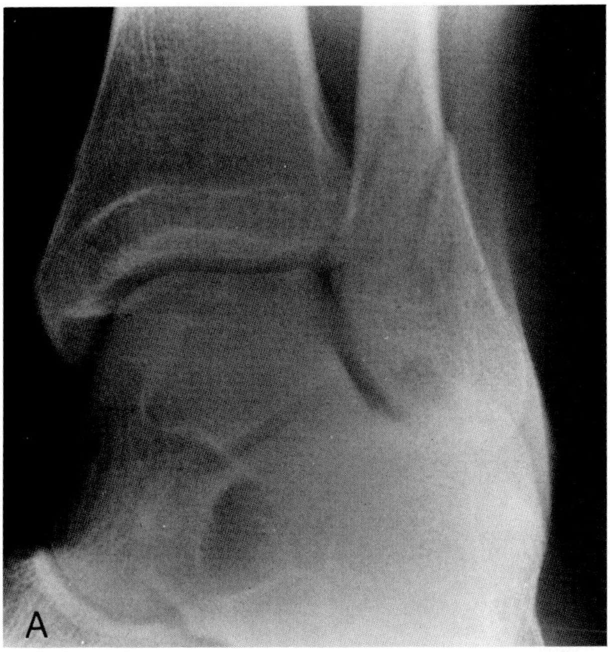

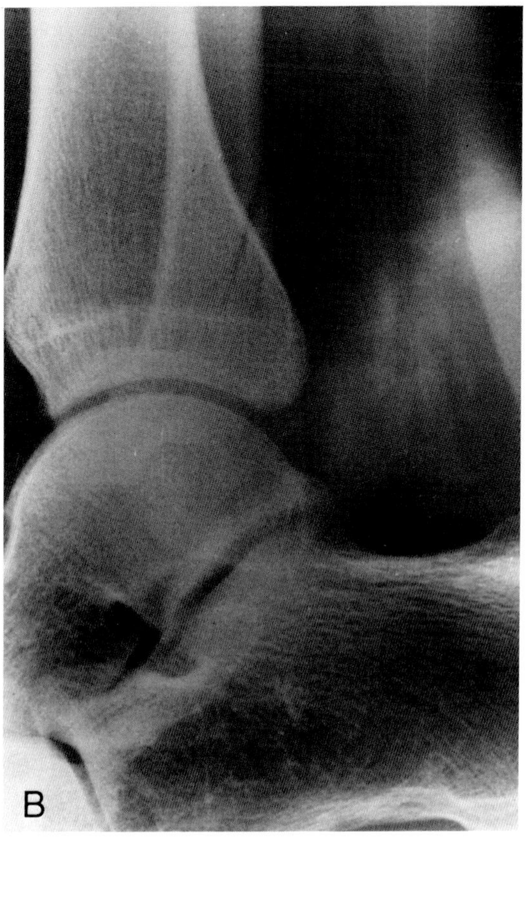

Fig. 13-3. Lateral malleolar fracture. (A) Mortise view. (B) Lateral view.

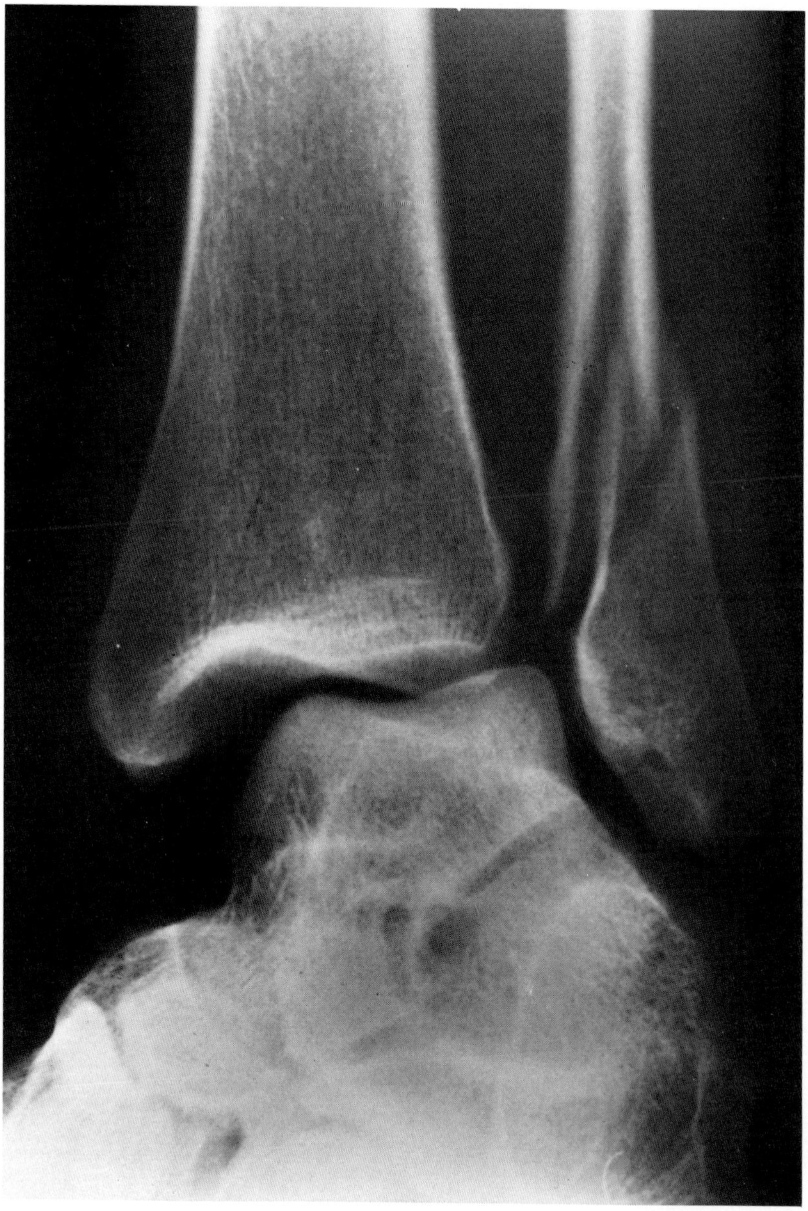

Fig. 13-4. Lateral malleolar fracture with deltoid ligament tear. Note the increased space between medial malleolus and the talus.

Bimalleolar Fracture

MECHANISM

Varying mechanisms of injury involving significant force.

CLINICAL PRESENTATION

Pain, swelling, and deformity if the fracture is displaced.

ROENTGENOGRAMS

AP, lateral, and mortise views (Fig. 13-5) should be obtained.

COMPLICATIONS

Skin problems.

TREATMENT

Anatomic reduction, immobilization in long leg plaster, and admission to the hospital for observation. Open reduction and internal fixation is necessary if anatomic reduction cannot be obtained by closed means.

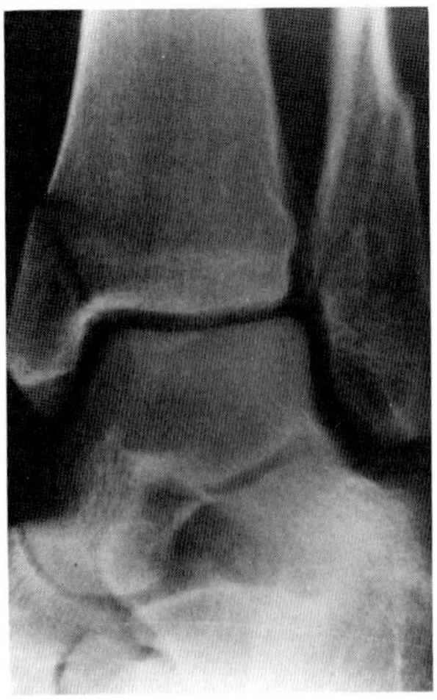

Fig. 13-5. Bimalleolar fracture. Fracture of both the medial and lateral malleolus renders the ankle joint unstable.

Maisonneuve Fracture

Isolated fracture of the fibular occurs almost exclusively after a direct blow. Any fracture of the fibula above the level of the tibial plafond should be considered part of an injury complex involving disruption of the syndesmosis and either ligamentous or bony injury to the medial side of the joint.

MECHANISM

An external rotation force transmitted to the proximal fibula after the syndesmosis is torn.

CLINICAL PRESENTATION

The primary complaint is ankle pain and swelling. Direct tenderness is present over the fibular fracture, which may be as proximal as the fibular neck. The fibular fracture may be occult, and only recognized on direct palpation.

ROENTGENOGRAMS

AP, lateral, and mortise views of the ankle will reveal widening of the mortise or a medial malleolar fracture. The distal fibula is intact. Roentgenograms of the entire leg should be obtained to reveal the proximal fibular fracture. A syndesmosis tear is likely if there is more than 5 mm of space between the tibia and the fibula on the mortise view or less than 10 mm over lap of the fibula and tibia on the AP view (Fig. 13-6).

COMPLICATIONS

Failure to recognize and treat the widening of the mortise will ultimately result in degenerative arthritis of the ankle.

TREATMENT

Open reduction and internal fixation are necessary.

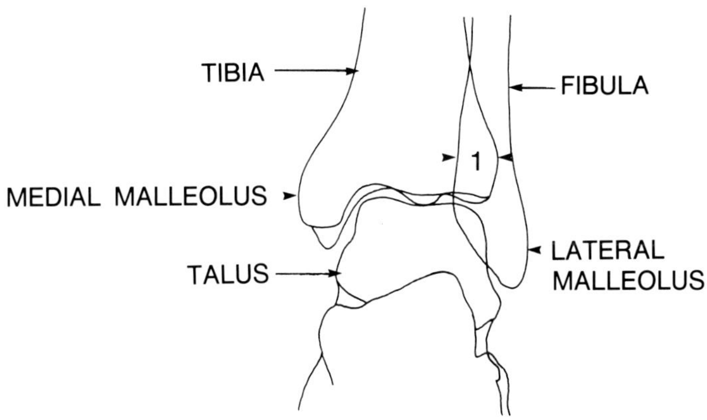

Fig. 13-6. The normal relationships between the tibia and fibula on the AP view should reveal an overlap of one cm. Overlap less than 10 mm may represent a disruption of the interosseous membrane.

Trimalleolar Fracture-Dislocation

MECHANISM

Trimalleolar fractures are produced by significant force. The injury most often occurs when the foot is planted and the body continues forward over it.

CLINICAL PRESENTATION

The deformity is obvious. There is often significant swelling. The skin may be tented over the fractured bone ends.

ROENTGENOGRAMS

AP, lateral, and mortise views (Fig. 13-7) will reveal fractures of the medial, lateral malleoli, as well as the "posterior malleolus" (posterior lip of the tibia).

COMPLICATIONS

Damage to the skin is not frequent. Neurovascular problems are unusual, but can occur.

TREATMENT

Reduction of the dislocation is usually accomplished with gentle longitudinal traction on the calcaneus. A long-leg splint or Quigley's traction may be used if swelling precludes the application of the long-leg cast. Open reduction is often required.

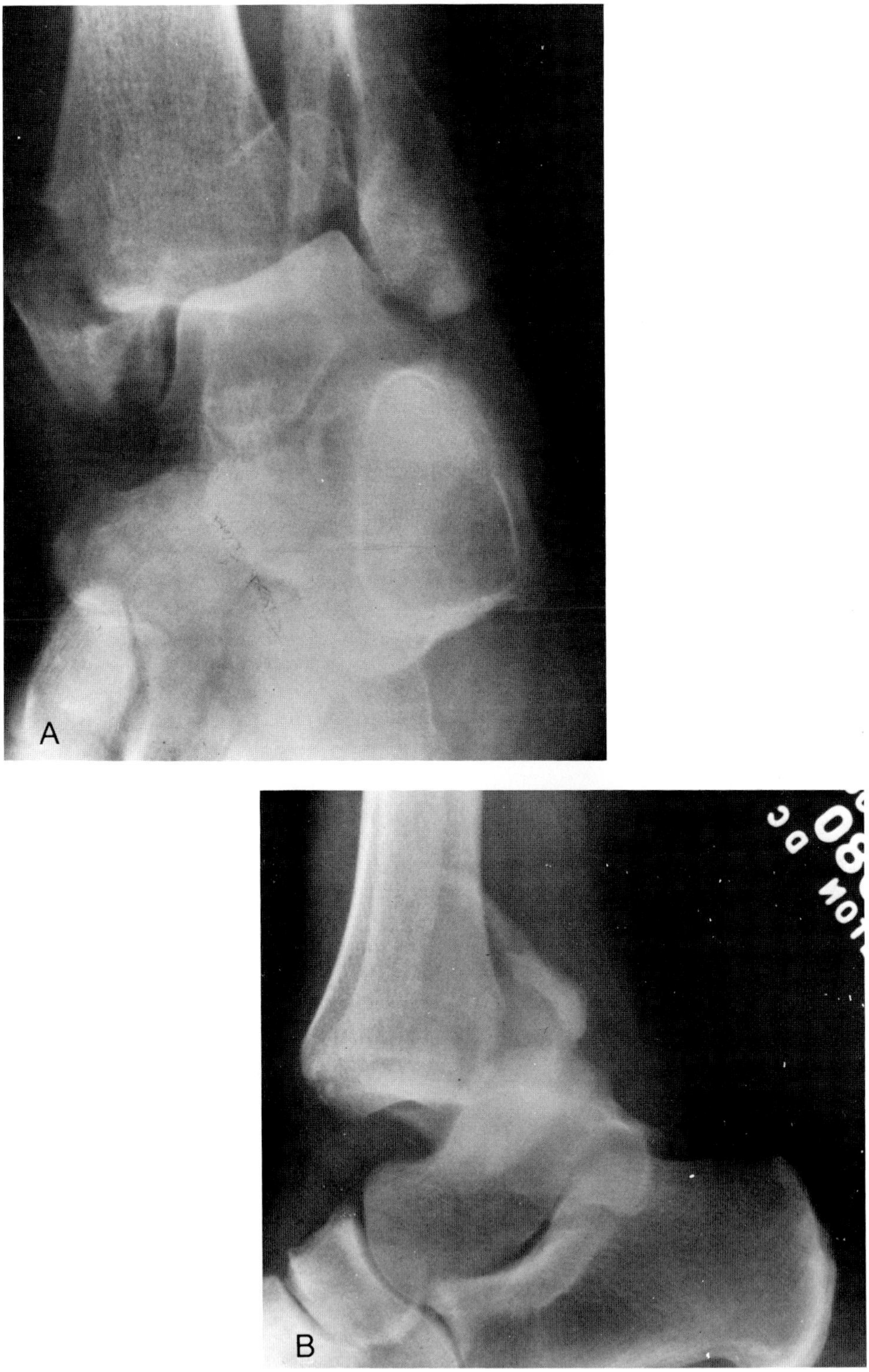

Fig. 13-7. Trimalleolar fracture dislocation. (A) AP view. (B) Lateral view. Note the talus is dislocated posteriorly.

Chip Fracture

Chip fractures may be seen at the insertion of the anterior capsule of the ankle into either the navicular or the talus.

MECHANISM

These fractures are usually avulsions of the capsular insertions. They occur with acute inversion and flexion injuries and are often associated with ankle sprains.

CLINICAL PRESENTATION

Acute swelling; tenderness of the foot. Ankle motion is painful. Point tenderness is present at the site of the avulsion.

ROENTGENOGRAMS

The lateral roentgenogram is the most valuable film. The AP and mortise should also be obtained to exclude other ankle injuries.

COMPLICATIONS

Rare.

TREATMENT

Treatment as for sprains.

Osteochondral Fracture

MECHANISM

Axial compression or forced dorsiflexion of the ankle, causing compression of the talus against the ankle mortise. The injury may not be recognized acutely and the patient will continue to complain of pain.

CLINICAL PRESENTATION

The patient may have vague symptoms of deep ankle pain that cannot be localized. This injury is often misdiagnosed as osteochondritis dissecans or "ankle sprain" because of the apparently negative roentgenograms.

ROENTGENOGRAMS

In addition to the routine AP, lateral and mortise views of the ankle, an AP of the foot in full plantar flexion is helpful in evaluating the dome of the talus. Tomograms are usually necessary.

COMPLICATIONS

Persistent pain. Late post-traumatic arthritis of the ankle.

TREATMENT

Immobilization in a short-leg walking cast may allow the fragments to heal. Frequently, a displaced fragment may require surgical excision.

Fractures of the Talus

Fractures of the talus often present as "ankle fractures." The talus is the keystone of the longitudinal arch of the foot. It supports and distributes the body weight and is the second most common tarsal bone to be fractured. The talus has an extensive articular surface (over 50%) and articulates with the tibia, fibula, calcaneus, and navicular. Because it has no muscle or tendonous attachment to carry vascular supply, it is highly susceptible to avascular necrosis following fracture. Open fracture of the talus is not infrequent. The most common talar fractures are the chip fracture (35%) and fracture of the talar neck (30%).

MECHANISM

Forced hyperextension of the foot and ankle. The neck is forced against the anterior tibia which acts as a fulcrum, resulting in fracture of the neck of the talus.

CLINICAL PRESENTATION

The patient presents with pain and swelling of the ankle. Any motion of the foot or ankle is greatly resisted. Tenderness is poorly localized.

ROENTGENOGRAMS

AP, lateral, and oblique roentgenograms (Fig. 13-8) of the foot are necessary.

COMPLICATIONS

Avascular necrosis and talar dislocation can occur.

TREATMENT

Reduction and immobilization in a long-leg cast, non weight-bearing. Open reduction is required if anatomic reduction cannot be obtained by closed manipulation.

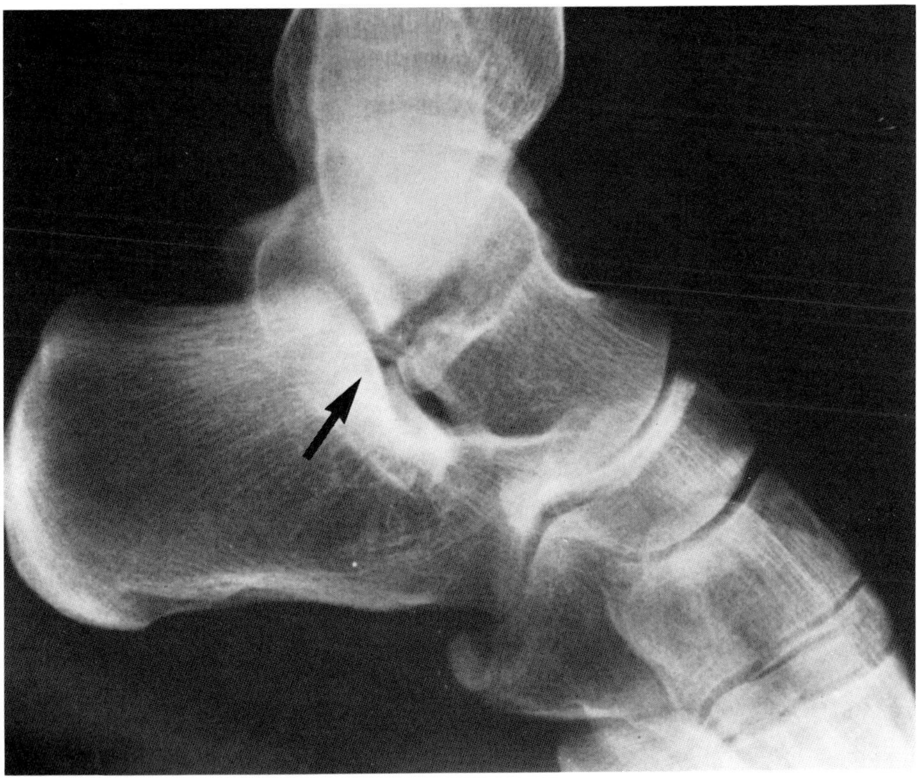

Fig. 13-8. Fracture of the neck of the talus. The fracture is best seen on the lateral view.

Subtalar Dislocation

MECHANISM

Severe trauma with the ankle in flexion and inversion. The dislocation is usually medial; 15 percent of patients do not have an associated fracture.

CLINICAL PRESENTATION

There is severe pain and swelling with gross deformity of the foot. The skin will be tented over the head of the talus. Neurovascular compromise may occur.

ROENTGENOGRAMS

AP, lateral, and oblique roentgenograms (Fig. 13-9) are needed to evaluate the position of the foot and possible fractures.

COMPLICATIONS

Avascular necrosis occurs in 10 to 15 percent of these patients.

TREATMENT

Reduction should be accomplished as soon as possible. General anesthesia may be required.

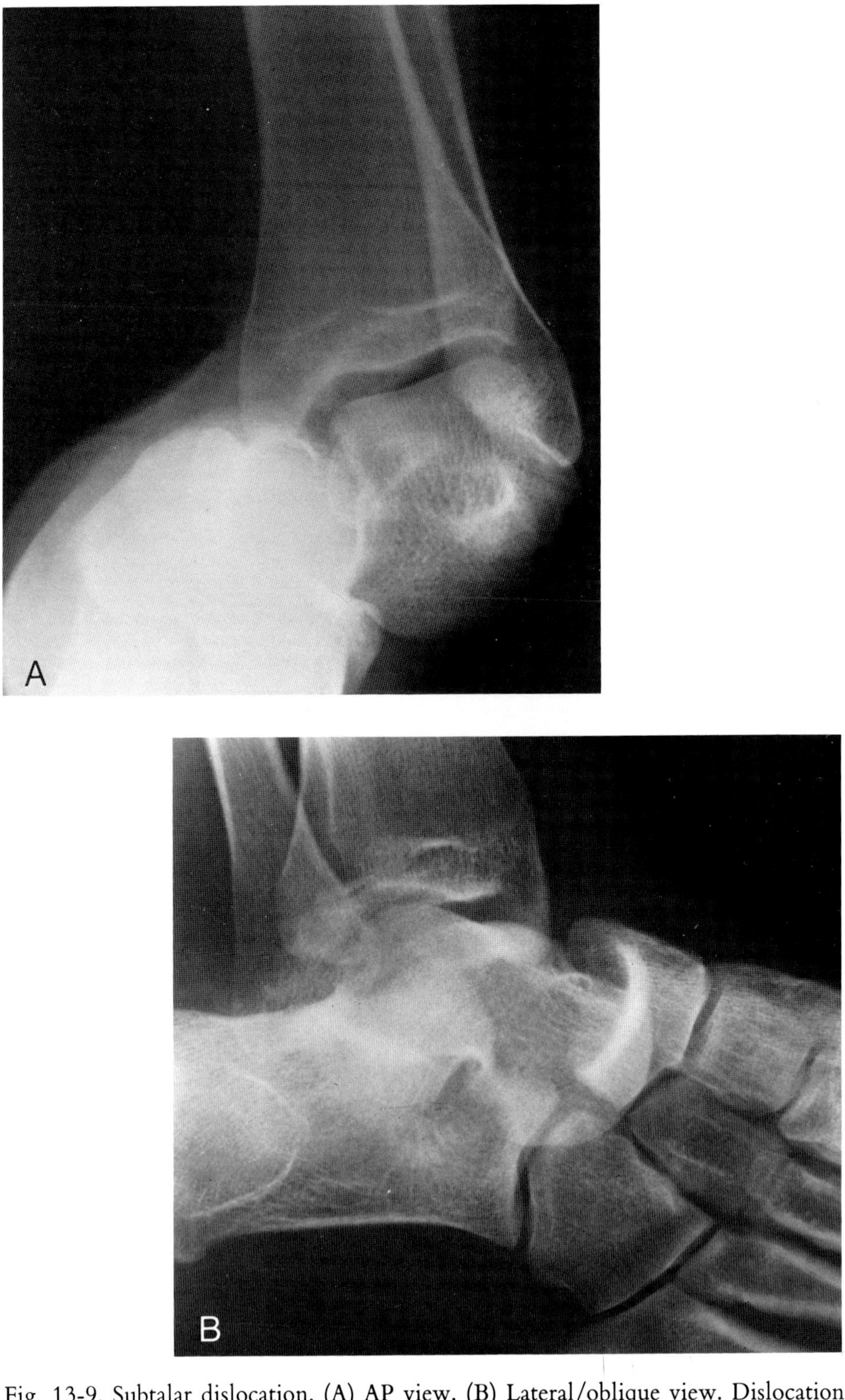

Fig. 13-9. Subtalar dislocation. (A) AP view. (B) Lateral/oblique view. Dislocation occurs at the subtalar joint. Notice that the talus is located within the ankle mortise.

14 The Foot

The foot is subject to both direct and indirect trauma. Adequate radiographic examination consists of three views: the AP (Fig. 14-1A), lateral (Fig. 14-1B), and oblique (Fig. 14-1C).

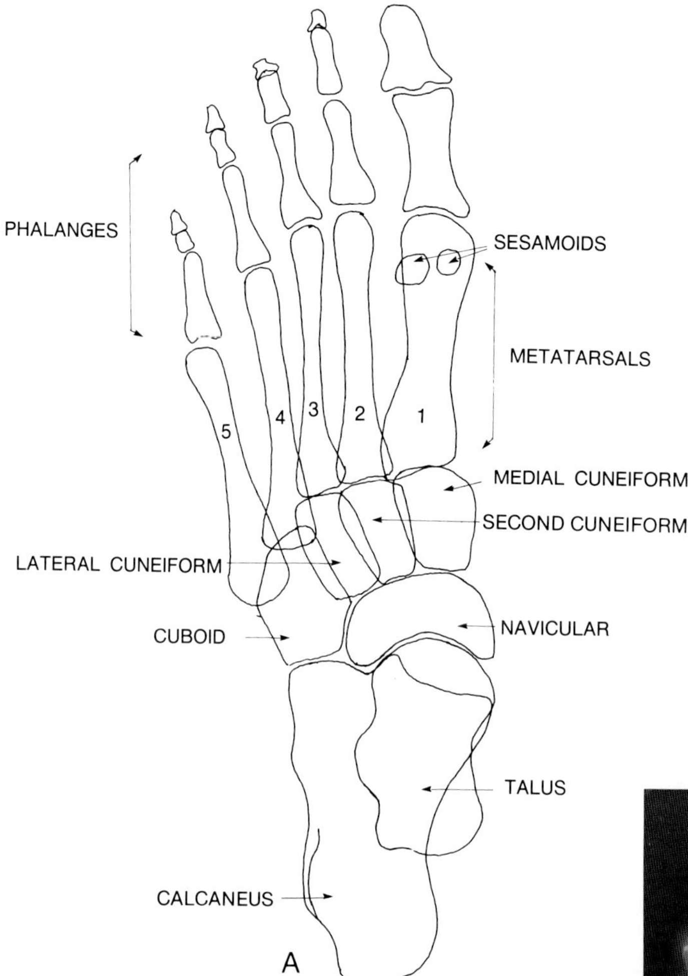

PHALANGES
SESAMOIDS
METATARSALS
5
4
3
2
1
MEDIAL CUNEIFORM
SECOND CUNEIFORM
LATERAL CUNEIFORM
CUBOID
NAVICULAR
TALUS
CALCANEUS

A

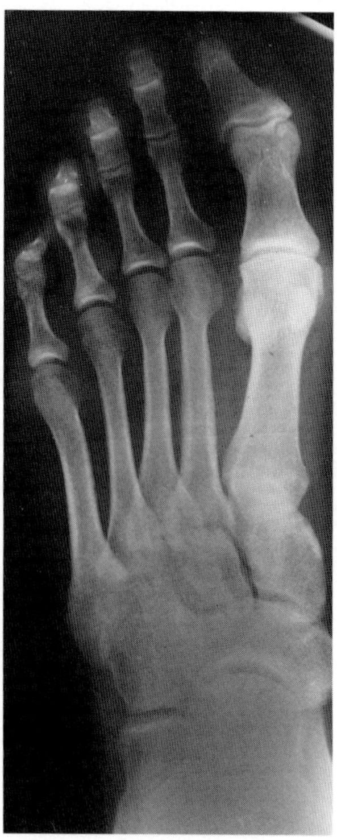

A

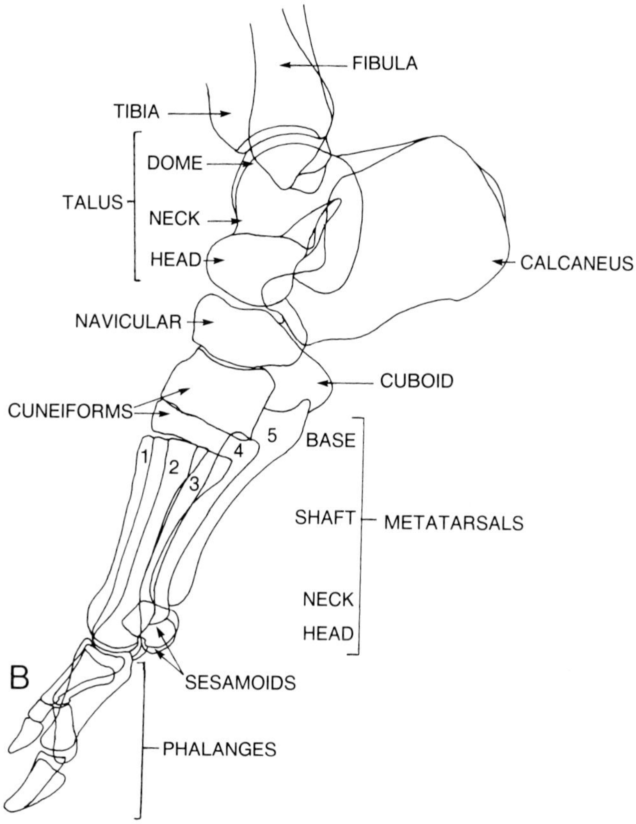

B

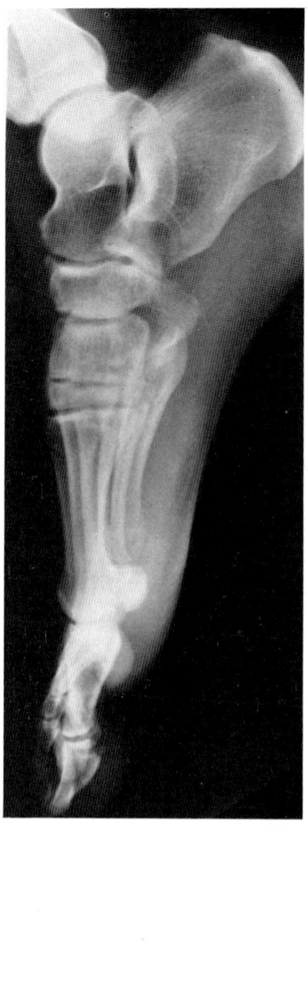

B

Fig. 14-1. (A) AP view of the foot — normal. (B) Lateral view of the foot — normal (Figure continues).

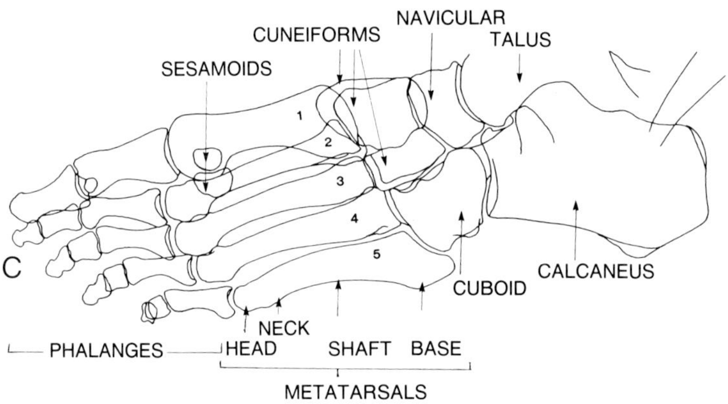

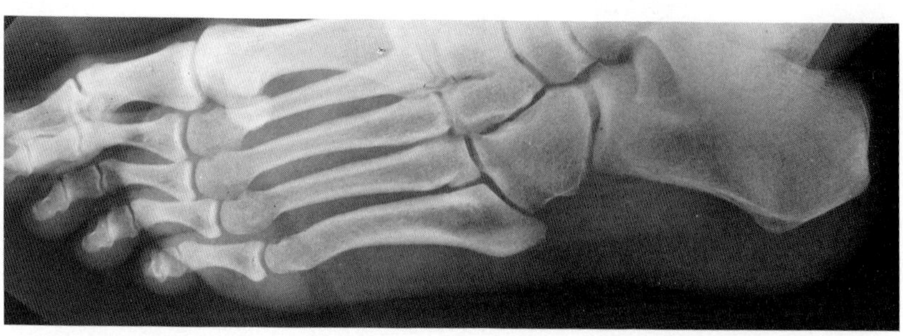

Fig. 14-1 (Continued). (C) Oblique view of the foot — normal.

Calcaneus Fractures

The calcaneus is the most frequently fractured tarsal bone. Adequate examination requires a special axial view (Fig. 14-2A) and a standard lateral view (Fig. 14-2B). Injuries to the calcaneus produce significant long-term disability.

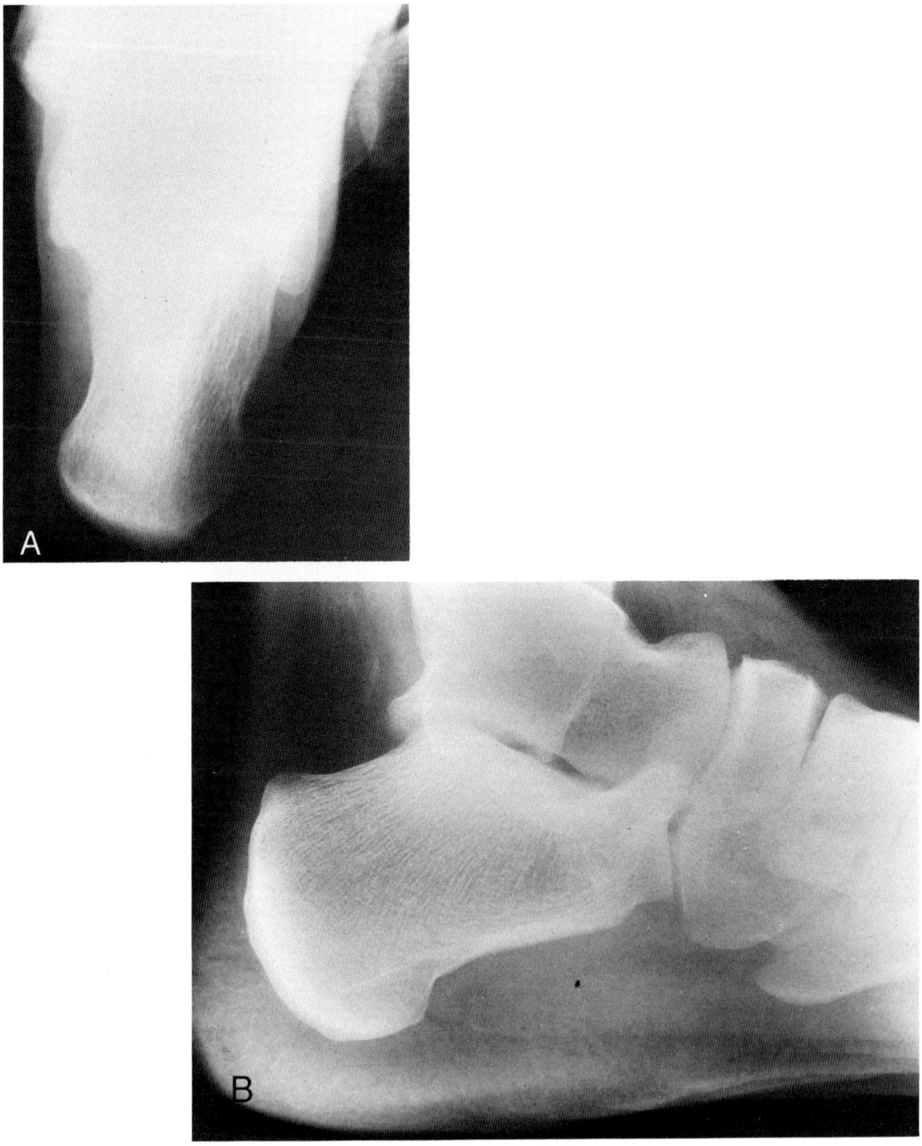

Fig. 14-2. (A) Axial view of the calcaneus — normal. (B) Lateral view of the calcaneus — normal.

MECHANISM

Usually a jump or a fall from a significant height. The calcaneus is crushed when the talus is driven down into the body.

CLINICAL PRESENTATION

The patient is not able to bear weight. The foot is swollen and tender and the heel may be widened.

ROENTGENOGRAMS

AP and lateral views of the foot (Fig. 14-4) and an axial view of the calcaneus should be obtained. Bohler's angle, connecting the highest points of the anterior process, posterior facet and calcaneal tuberosity, should be measured on the lateral. When the normal angle of 25 to 40 degrees is lost in severe crush injuries, the prognosis is poor.

COMPLICATIONS

Concomitant fracture of the lumbar spine occurs in 10 percent of patients, and other lower extremity fractures in 25 percent. Roentgenograms should be obtained of almost any area where the patient with calcaneal fracture has pain. Long-term sequellae include a widened, painful heel and subtalar arthritis.

TREATMENT

Elevation and immobilization in a bulky compressive dressing, with or without a splint. Early motion is helpful, but weight-bearing is not permitted for three months.

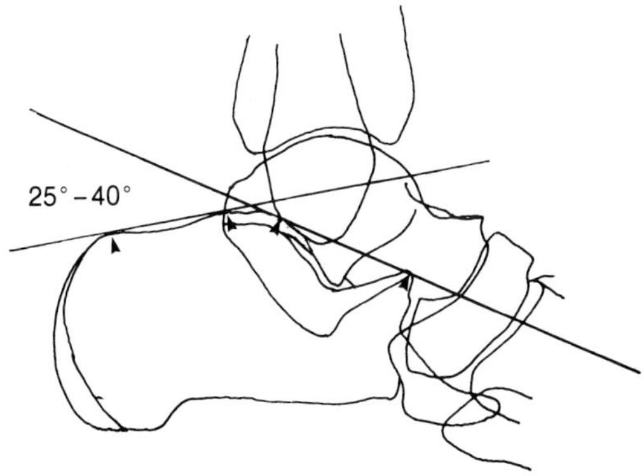

Fig. 14-3. Böhler's angle. The angle, should be in the range 25–40°.

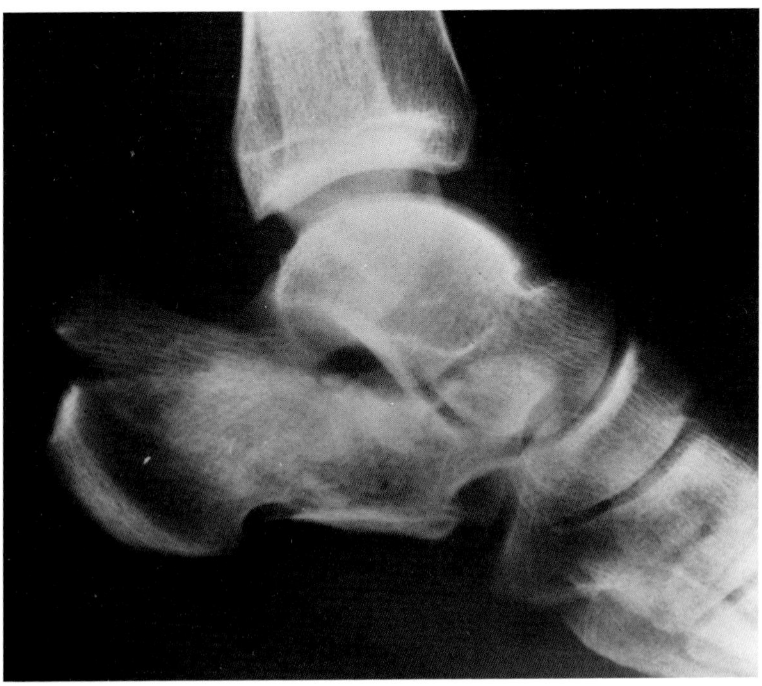

Fig. 14-4. Calcaneal fracture. Note the loss of Böhler's angle.

Tarsometatarsal Dislocations (Lisfranc)

MECHANISM

The most common mechanism of injury is a fall from a height or an automobile accident where the weight of the body is borne on the metatarsals with the foot in equinus (as when pressing on the brake pedal). The second mechanism is a twisting injury with the forefoot held fixed.

CLINICAL PRESENTATION

The patient has severe deformity of the foot with marked pain and swelling. There may be paresthesias and an absent or diminished dorsalis pedis pulse. The forefoot is shortened with prominence of the base of the fifth metatarsal.

ROENTGENOGRAMS

AP, lateral, and oblique roentgenograms should be obtained (Fig. 14-5). Multiple fractures of the bases of the metatarsals are equivalent to Lisfranc dislocation.

COMPLICATIONS

Posterior dislocation of the hip may be an associated injury. Vascular impairment and paresthesias are generally relieved by reduction of the dislocation.

TREATMENT

Reduction and internal fixation.

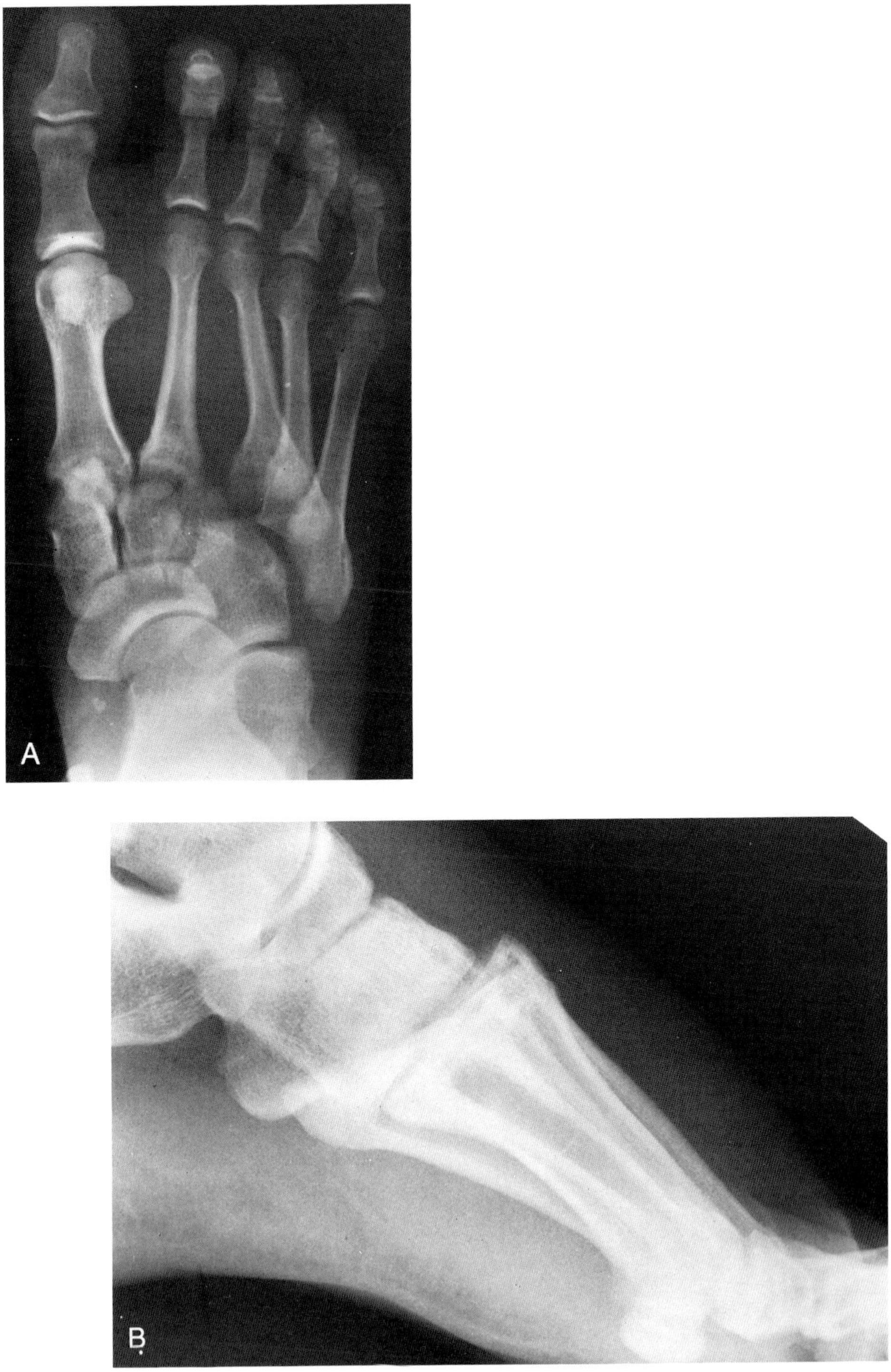

Fig. 14-5. Lisfrac fracture dislocation. (A) AP view. (B) Lateral view. The metatarsals have fractures and are dislocated from their normal alignment with the tarsal bones.

Metatarsal Fractures

MECHANISM

The metatarsal is subject to both direct and indirect trauma. Direct blows or a heavy object landing on the foot commonly produce fractures of the metatarsal neck or distal shaft. The indirect trauma of forceful muscle pulls causes avulsion fractures.

CLINICAL PRESENTATION

Pain, swelling, and tenderness are present over the fracture site. Ambulation is painful.

ROENTGENOGRAMS

AP, lateral, and oblique views (Fig. 14-6) of the foot should be obtained.

COMPLICATIONS

Severe swelling may accompany a crush injury, requiring hospitalization for observation and elevation.

TREATMENT

Symptomatic treatment with crutches, walking cast, or hard-soled shoe with weight-bearing as tolerated.

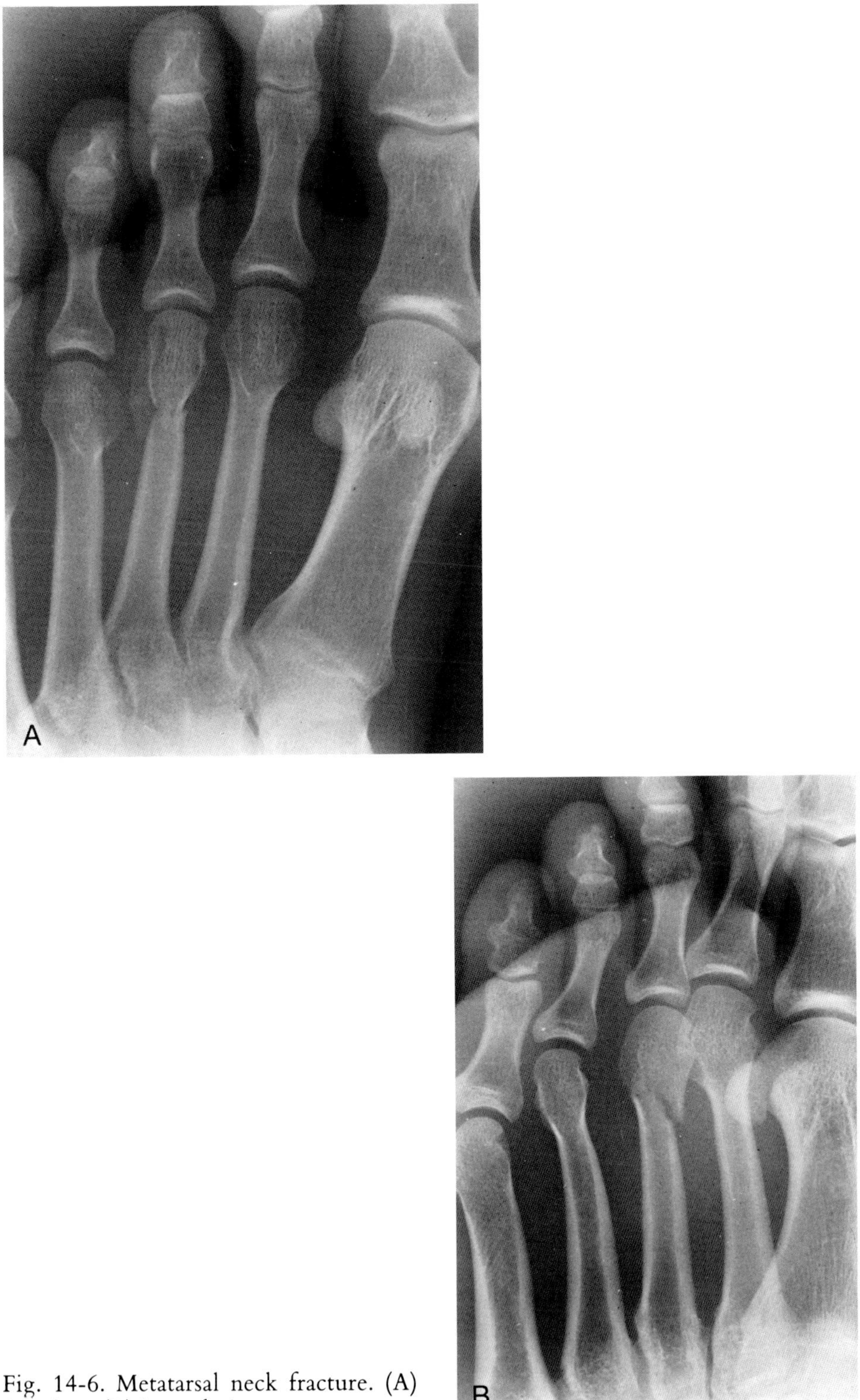

Fig. 14-6. Metatarsal neck fracture. (A) AP view. (B) Lateral view.

Stress Fracture

MECHANISM

Stress fractures of the shaft of the metatarsal are produced by repeated or unaccustomed stresses. There is a high incidence in military recruits ("march fractures") and runners.

CLINICAL PRESENTATION

Pain and tenderness over the metatarsal shafts should suggest a stress fracture. There may be a history of repeated stresses or a change in activity. The patient may present initially with unexplained pain in the forefoot, little ecchymosis or swelling, and a negative roentgenogram. Follow-up films in three to four weeks will show callus and/or periosteal thickening. Bone scan will confirm the diagnosis, but is not routinely indicated.

ROENTGENOGRAMS

Initial roentgenograms are negative. Periosteal reaction may be seen in three to four weeks (Fig. 14-7). Technetium bone scan is positive.

COMPLICATIONS

Misdiagnosis.

TREATMENT

Symptomatic treatment.

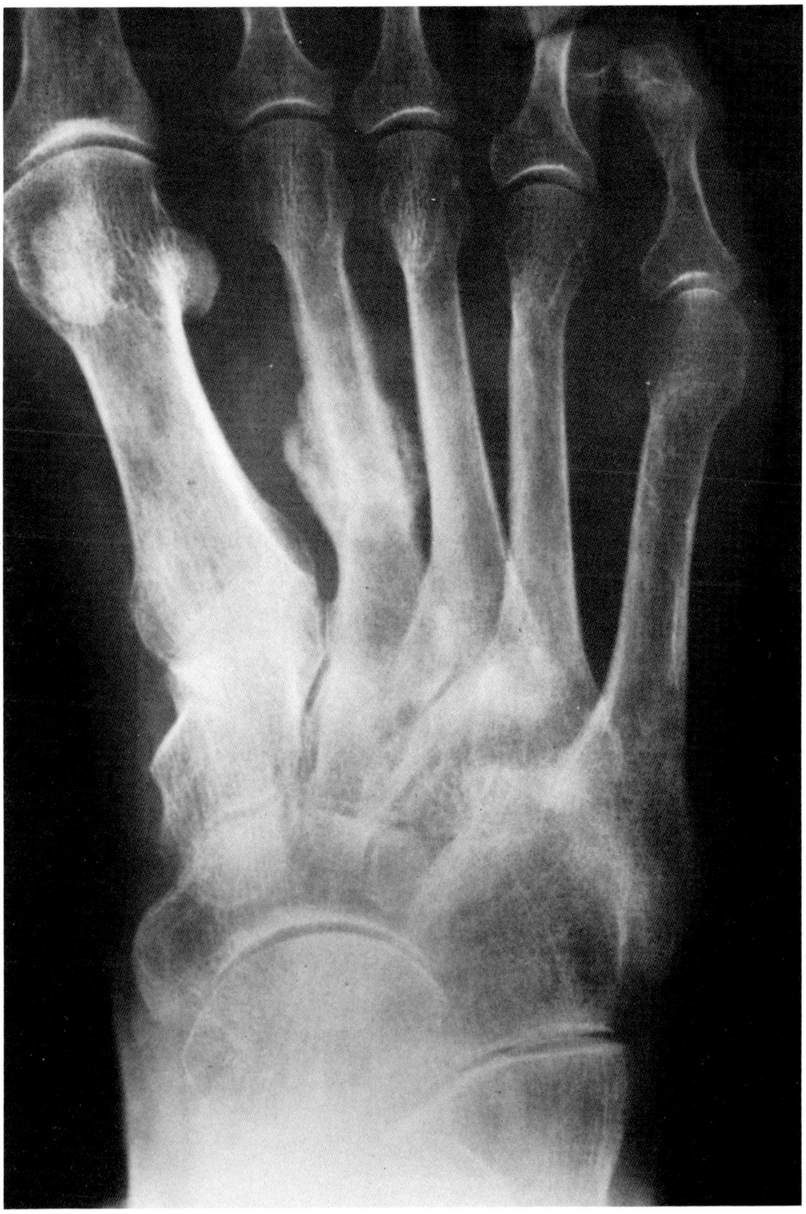

Fig. 14-7. Stress fracture of the second metatarsal. Periosteal reaction is present.

Jones Fracture

MECHANISM

Injury to the base of the fifth metatarsal is the most common metatarsal fracture. It results from a forceful contraction of the peroneus brevis in response to acute inversion and plantar flexion.

CLINICAL PRESENTATION

The patient gives a history of twisting the foot or turning suddenly. Pain and swelling are localized at the base of the fifth metatarsal.

ROENTGENOGRAMS

AP, lateral, and oblique films of the foot will reveal the injury (Fig. 14-8).

COMPLICATIONS

This fracture is often missed when ankle films are ordered and reported to be normal.

TREATMENT

Symptomatic treatment with a soft dressing, walking cast, adhesive strapping or hard-soled shoe. Weight-bearing as tolerated.

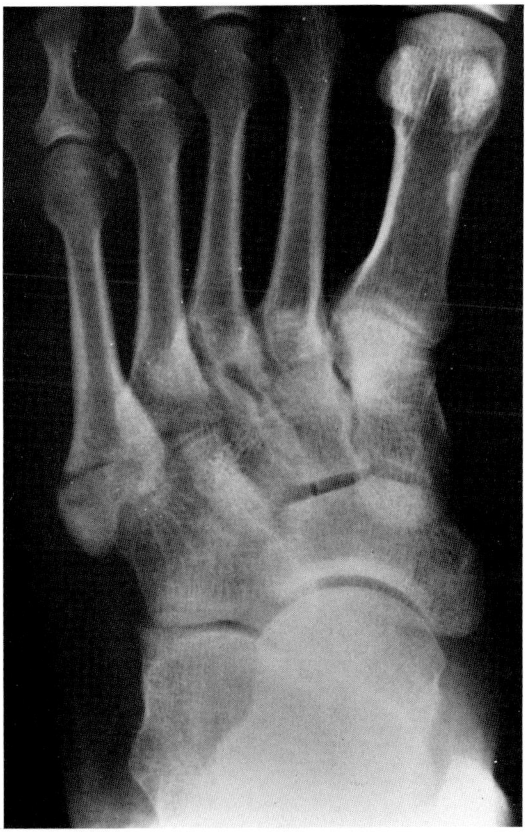

Fig. 14-8. Jones fracture (base of the 5th metatarsal).

Fractures of the Phalanges

MECHANISM

Fractures of the phalanges are usually the result of direct trauma—either an object falling on the toe or striking the toe while walking.

CLINICAL PRESENTATION

The toe or toes are swollen and tender. Subungual hematoma may be present.

ROENTGENOGRAMS

AP and lateral roentgenograms (Fig. 14-9) should be obtained. An oblique view may give additional information.

COMPLICATIONS

Dislocations may occur at the interphalangeal or metatarsophalangeal level.

TREATMENT

Fractures may be reduced, "buddy taped" to an adjacent toe, padded, and treated in a hard-soled shoe. Dislocations should be reduced with traction under the appropriate anesthesia. Once reduced, these injuries are usually stable and are treated like a fracture with "buddy taping" and a hard-soled shoe.

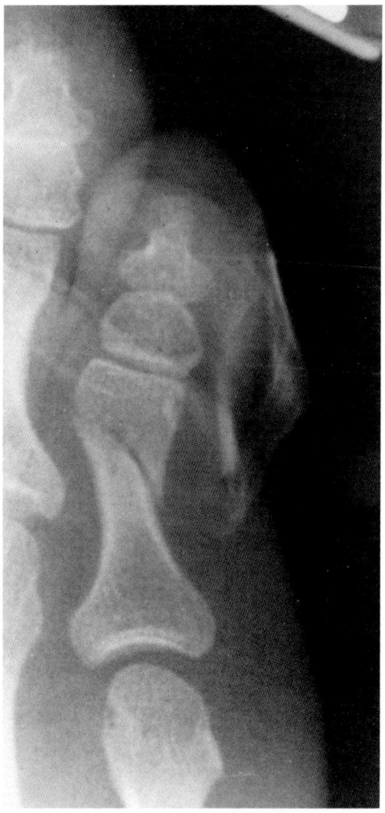

Fig. 14-9. Proximal phalanx fracture, fifth toe.

INDEX

Page numbers followed by an *f* indicate figures; those follwed by a *t* indicate tables.

Ace bandage, 241
Acetabulum
  anteroposterior view of, 174f, 186f
  dislocation of, 180, 181f
  fracture of, 182, 183f
  lateral view of, 187f
Acromioclavicular joint
  anteroposterior view of, 58f
  axillary view of, 59f
  dislocation of, 66, 67f
Acromion
  anteroposterior view of, 58f
  axillary view of, 59f
Adductor tubercle
  anteroposterior view of, 205f
  lateral view of, 206f
Ankle
  anteroposterior view of, 239f
  bimalleolar fracture of, 245, 245f
  chip fracture of, 250
  injuries of, 237–254
    clinical presentation of, 238
    mechanism of, 237
  lateral malleolar fracture of, 242, 243f, 244f
  Maisonneuve fracture of, 246, 247f
  Mortise view of, 240f
  osteochondral fracture of, 251
  sprain of, 241
  subtalar dislocation of, 254, 255f
  trimalleolar fracture dislocation of, 248, 249f
  "twisted," 238
Anterior arch, flexion fracture of, 18
Articular facet
  inferior
    anteroposterior view of, 38f
    oblique view of, 14f
  lateral view of, 39f
  superior
    anteroposterior view of, 38f
    oblique view of, 14f
Atlanto-axial (C1-C2) instability, of cervical spine, 30, 31f
Automobile accident, hangman's fracture and, 22
Avascular necrosis, talar fracture and, 252

Barton's fracture, 124, 125f
Basion, odontoid process and, 16f
  occipital-atlanto instability and, 29f
Bennett's fracture dislocation, 148, 149f
Bimalleolar fracture, 245, 245f
Böhler's angle, calcaneal fracture and, 263f
Bowman's angle, 88, 89f
Brown-Sequard syndrome, 32
"Burst" fracture, of cervical spine, 24, 25f

Calcaneous
  anteroposterior view of, 232f, 239f
  axial view of, 261f
  Böhler's angle of, 263f
  fracture of, 261–263
  lateral view of, 239f, 261f
  oblique view of, 260f

Capitate
anteroposterior view of, 114f, 140f
lateral view of, 115f, 141f
oblique view of, 116f, 141f
Capitellum, fracture of, 86
Capitellus, fracture of, radial head fracture and, 92
Capitolunate angle, 118, 119f
Carpal, dislocation of, 134, 134f
Cauda-equina injury, 42
Cervical spine
anterior dislocation of, 30
anterior subluxation of, 15, 15f
anteroposterior view of, 11–12, 12f
atlanto-axial (C10C2) instability of, 30, 31f
"burst" fracture of, 24, 25f
"clay-shoveler's" fracture of, 26, 27f
dislocation of, 12, 32, 33f
hangman fracture of, 22, 23f
horizontal translation of, 15f
injuries of, 11
instability of, 17, 17f
Jefferson fracture of, 18, 19f
lateral relationships of, 16f
lateral view of, 12, 13f, 15
lower
dislocation of, 32, 33f
subluxation of, 32
oblique view of, 12, 14f
occipital-atlanto (C1) instability of, 28, 29f
odontoid fracture of, 20–21, 21f
open-mouth view of, 12, 13f, 17
posterior dislocation of, 30
rotatory subluxation of, 30
strain on, 34
subluxation of, 32
teardrop fracture of, 24, 25f
Chance fracture, of thoracolumbar spine, 50, 51f
Chip fracture
of ankle, 250
of talus, 252
Clavicle
anteroposterior view of, 36f, 58f
axillary view of, 59f
fracture of, 62, 63f
lateral view of, 37f
"Clay-shoveler's" fracture, of cervical spine, 26, 27f
Coccyx, anteroposterior view of, 174f
Collar
cervical, 34
Philadelphia, for odontoid fractures, 21
soft, for "clay-shovelers" fracture, 26
Collateral ligament, injury to, 229
Colle's fracture, of wrist, 120, 121f
Compression fracture, of thoracolumbar spine, 44, 45f
Coracoid process
anteroposterior view of, 58f
axillary view of, 59f
fracture of, dislocated shoulder and, 70
Cruciate ligament, injury to, 230
Cuboid
anteroposterior view of, 239f, 258f
lateral view of, 239f, 259f
oblique view of, 260f
Cuneiform
anteroposterior view of, 239f, 258f
lateral view of, 239f, 259f
oblique view of, 260f

Deltoid ligament, lateral malleolar fracture and, 242, 244f
Disc, ruptured, 54
Dislocation
of acetabulum, 180, 181f
acromioclavicular, 66, 67f
of carpal, 134, 134f
dorsal, 166, 166f, 167f
of elbow, 94, 94f, 95f
of hip, 180, 181f
interphalangeal, 166
anteroposterior view of, 166f
lateral view of, 167f
oblique view of, 167f
of knee, 224, 225f
Lisfranc, 264, 265f
of lunate, 135, 135f
metacarpophalangeal, 162
anteroposterior view of, 163f
lateral view of, 164f
oblique view of, 165f
of patella, 226, 227f

perilunate, 136, 136f, 137f
of shoulder
anterior, 69–70, 69f, 70f, 71f
posterior, 72–73, 72f, 73f
sternoclavicular, 68
of subtalar joint, 252, 253f
of tarsometatarsal joint, 264, 265f
volar, 158, 169f

Elbow
anterior dislocation of, 96
anteroposterior view of, 84f
"carrying angle" of, 83
dislocation of, 86, 94, 94f, 95f
anterior, 96
anteroposterior view of, 94f
lateral view of, 95f
equilateral triangle of, 86, 87f
"fat pad" sign of, 86, 87f
fracture dislocation of, 105f
lateral view of, 85f
oblique view of, 85f
radial capitellar alignment of, 86f

"Fat pad" sign, 86, 87f
Femur
anteroposterior view of, 174f, 186f, 205f
fracture of, 204–208
anteroposterior view of, 217f
lateral view of, 217f
lateral view of, 187f, 206f–207f
neck of, fracture of, 189–190
shaft of, fracture of, 209f
subcapital fracture of, 191f
supracondylar fracture of, 206, 217f
Fibula
anteroposterior view of, 205f, 232f
fracture of, 231–234, 234f, 235f
lateral view of, 206f, 233f
Finger, -hand alignment of, 142, 142f, 143f
Foot
anteroposterior view of, 258f
injuries of, 257–272
lateral view of, 259f
oblique view of, 260f
Forearm
anteroposterior view of, 102f
distal, fracture of, 110
fracture of, 101–112
Galleazzi fracture dislocation of, 111–112, 111f, 112f
lateral view of, 103f
middle, fracture of, 110
Fracture
angulation, 7, 7f
avulsion, 5
Barton's, 124, 125f
"buddy strapped," 272
of calcaneous, 261–262, 263f
chance, of thoracolumbar spine, 50, 51f
chip, 250, 252
of clavicle, 62, 63f
closed, 2, 3f
Colle's, 120, 121f
comminuted, 3, 3f
compression, of thoracolumbar spine, 44, 45f
dislocation, *see* Fracture-dislocation
displacement, 7, 7f
extra-articular, of first metacarpal, 151, 151f
Galleazzi dislocation, 111–112, 111f, 112f
of greater tuberosity, 79f
of hamate, 131f
hangman's, 22, 23f
of humerus, 76–80
Jefferson, 18, 19f
Jones, 270, 271f
of lunate, 129
Maisonneuve, 246
Monteggia, 104, 105f
mallet finger, 156, 157f
of metatarsals, 266, 267f
nightstick, of ulna, 108, 109f
oblique, 4, 4f
of odontoid, 20–21, 21f
of olecranon, 90, 91f
open, 2, 2f
ostechondral, 251
of patella, 218, 219f
of phalanges, 272, 273f
of proximal humerus, 78
of radius, 92, 93f
Rolando, 150
of scaphoid, 126–128, 126f, 127f

Fracture *(Continued)*
of scapula, 64, 65f
shear, 129
Smith's, 122, 123f
spiral, 4, 4f
stellate, 4
stress, 268, 269f
subluxation, 5
supracondylar
of femur, 216, 217f
of humerus, 88, 89f
terminology of, 1–7
of tibial plateau, 220, 221f
transverse, 3, 3f
of transverse process, 48, 49f
of triquetrium, 131f
valgus alignment, 6, 6f
varus alignment, 5, 5f
volar avulsion, 158, 158f
volvar, 125f
wedge, of thoracolumbar spine, 46, 47f
Fracture-dislocation, 5
Bennett's, 148, 149f
of elbow, 105f
of metacarpal, 148, 149f
of thoracolumbar spine, 44, 45f
trimalleolar, 248, 249f

Gamekeeper's thumb, 152, 153f
Gelo boot, 241
Glenohumeral joint
dislocation of
anterior, 69–70, 69f–71f
"ice-cream cone" appearance of, 72
posterior, 72–73, 72f–73f
separation of, 66, 67f
Glenoid cavity
anteroposterior view of, 58f
axillary view of, 59f
fracture of, dislocated shoulder and, 70
Greater trochanter
anteroposterior view of, 174f, 186f, 195f
fracture of, 195, 195f
lateral view of, 187f

"Halo," skeletal fixation with, 18
Hamate
anteroposterior view of, 114f, 140f
fracture of, 131f
lateral view of, 115f, 141f
oblique view of, 116f, 141f
Hand
anteroposterior view of, 140f
-finger alignment, 143f
fracture of, radial head fracture and, 92
lateral view of, 141f
oblique view of, 141f
Hangman's fracture, of cervical spine, 22, 23f
Hemarthrosis, elbow fracture and, 86
Hip
anterior dislocation of, 200, 201f
anteroposterior view of, 186f
central fracture of, 182, 183f
dislocation of, 199
anterior, 200, 201f
posterior, 202, 203f
extracapsular fracture of, 192
fracture of
classical position in, 189f
intracapsular, 189–190
intertrochanteric fracture of, 193f, 194f
lateral view of, 187f
posterior dislocation of, 202, 203f
posterior fracture dislocation of, 180, 181f
Shenton's line of, 185, 188f
subcapital fracture of, 191f
subtrochanteric fracture of, 198
Humerus
anteroposterior view of, 58f, 76f, 79f
aseptic necrosis of, 78
axillary view of, 59f, 79f
condyles of, fracture of, 86
fracture of, 86
greater tuberosity of, fracture of, 79f
lateral view of, 77f
proximal, fracture of, 78
radiography of, 76f
shaft, fracture of, 80, 81f
supracondylar fracture of, 88, 89f
surgical neck of, fracture of, 79f

Iliac crest, anteroposterior view of, 174f
Iliac wing, anteroposterior view of, 174f
Ilium
anteroposterior view of, 174f, 186f
lateral view of, 187f

Interosseous membrane
  anteroposterior view of, 232f
  disruption of, 247f
Intervertebral disc
  anteroposterior view of, 12f
  lateral view of, 13f, 16f, 39f
  oblique view of, 14f
Intervertebral foramen, lateral view of, 39f
Ischium
  anteroposterior view of, 174f, 186f
  lateral view of, 187f

Jefferson fracture, 18, 19f
Joint, fluid in, "fat pad" sign of, 87f
Jones fracture, of fifth metatarsal, 270, 271f

Kienböck's disease, 129
Knee
  anteroposterior view of, 212f
  dislocation of, 224, 225f
  injuries of, 211–230
  intercondylar view of, 215f
  lateral view of, 213f
  "locking" of, 228
  oblique view of, 214f
  patellar view of, 215f
  popping of, 226
  soft tissue injur about, 228–230
  sunrise view of, 215f
  tunnel view of, 215f

Lamina
  anteroposterior view of, 36f, 38f
  lateral view of, 37f, 39f
Lateral malleolus, 242
  fracture of, 243f, 244f
    with deltoid ligament tear, 244f
Lesser trochanter
  anteroposterior view of, 197f
  fracture of, 196, 197f
  subtrochanteric fracture of, 198
Lisfranc dislocation, 264, 265f
Lumbar spine
  anteroposterior view of, 38, 38f, 174f
  chance fracture of, 50, 51f
  herniated nucleus pulposus of, 54
  lateral view of, 38, 39f, 40f
  oblique view of, 40f
  ruptured disc of, 54
  spondylolisthesis of, 52, 53f
  "spot" lateral view of, 38, 41f
  strain of, 54
  transverse process fracture of, 48, 49f
  wedge fracture of, 46, 47f
Lunate
  anteroposterior view of, 114f, 140f
  dislocation of, 135, 135f
  fracture of, 129
  lateral view of, 141f, 155f
  oblique view of, 116f, 141f
  osteonecrosis of, 129

Maisonneuve fracture, 246
Malleolus
  anteroposterior view of, 232f
  lateral
    fracture of, 245f
      with deltoid ligament tear, 244f
    lateral view of, 243f
    Mortise view of, 243f
  medial
    fracture of, 245f
    Maisonneuve fracture and, 246
Mallet finger, 156, 157f
Menisci ligament, injury to, 228
Metacarpals
  alignment of, 142, 142f
  anteroposterior view of, 114f, 140f, 144f
  Boxer's fracture of, 144, 146f, 147f
  fifth, fracture of, 144, 147f
  first
    extra-articular fracture of, 151, 151f
    Gamekeeper's fracture of, 152, 153f
    "T" fracture of, 150
    "Y" fracture of, 150
  fracture of
    anteroposterior view of, 145f, 146f
    Bennett's fracture dislocation of, 148, 149f
    Boxer's, 147f
    clinical presentation of, 142
    complications of, 144
    dislocation of, 148, 149f
    fracture dislocation of, 148, 149f
    lateral view of, 145f, 147f
    mechanism of, 142

Metacarpals *(Continued)*
oblique view of, 145f, 147f
Rolando fracture of, 150
roentgenograms of, 144
treatment of, 144
lateral view of, 115f, 141f, 144f
oblique view of, 116f, 141f, 144f
-phalanges dislocation, 162, 163f 165f
third, fracture of, 145f
Metatarsals
anteroposterior view of, 258f, 267f
fracture of, 266, 267f
Jones fracture of, 270, 271f
lateral view of, 259f, 267f
oblique view of, 260f
stress fracture of, 268, 269f
Monteggia fracture, 104, 105f

Navicular
anteroposterior view of, 239f, 258f
lateral view of, 239f
oblique view of, 260f
Neck, hyperextension of, 34
Neural arch, fracture of, 22
Night stick fracture, of ulna, 108, 109f
Nucleus pulposus, hernia of, 54

Obturator foramen, anteroposterior view of, 174f
Occipital-atlanto (Cl) instability, of cervical spine, 28, 29f
Odontoid process
anteroposterior view of, 12f
avulsion of, 20, 20f
base of, fracture of, 29, 20f
body of, fracture of, 29, 20f
fracture of, 20–21, 21f
Jefferson fracture and, 18
open-mouthed view of, 21f
lateral view of, 13f, 16f
oblique view of, 14f
Olecranon
fossa, anteroposterior view of, 84f
fracture of, 86, 90, 91f
Osseous ring, Jefferson fracture of, 18, 19f
Osteochondral fracture, 251
patellar dislocation and, 226, 227f
Osteonecrosis, 129

Pain, low back, 54
Paraplegia, thoracolumbar fracture dislocation and, 42
Pars interarticularis, fracture of, 53f
Patella
anteroposterior view of, 205f
dislocation of, 226, 227f
fracture of, 218, 219f
lateral view of, 206f
Pelvis
anteroposterior view of, 174f, 183f
complex fracture of, 177f, 178
fracture of, 176
complex, 177f, 178
injury of, causes of, 173
Phalanges
injury of, 154–160
of foot
anteroposterior view of, 258f
fracture of, 272, 273f
lateral view of, 259f
oblique view of, 260f
of hand
anteroposterior view of, 140f, 161f
crushing injury of, 155f
distal, fracture of, 154, 155f
dorsal dislocation of, 166, 166f, 167f
lateral view of, 141f
oblique view of, 141f
of foot, fracture of, 272, 273f
middle, fracture of, 159
proximal, fracture of, 160, 161f
volar avulsion of, 158, 158f
volar dislocation of, 168, 169f
Philadelphia hand collar, for odontoid fractures, 21
Pisiform
anteroposterior view of, 114f, 140f
lateral view of, 115f, 141f
oblique view of, 116f, 141f
Pubic ramus
anteroposterior view of, 186f
fracture of, 179, 179f
inferior, anteroposterior view of, 174f
lateral view of, 187f
superior, anteroposterior view of, 174f

Pubis, anteroposterior view of, 174f

Quadriceps muscle, petallar fracture and, 218, 219f

Radius
  anterior dislocation of, 96
  Colles' fracture of, 113
  capitellar alignment of, 86f
  deviation of, 118, 118f
  distal, Barton's fracture of, 124, 125f
  fracture dislocation of, Galleazzi, 111–112, 111f, 112f
  fracture of, and ulna, 106, 107f
  Galleazzi fracture dislocation of, 111–112, 111f, 112f
  head of
    anteroposterior view of, 98f
    dislocation of, 86, 97, 98f
    oblique view of, 99f
  posterior dislocation of, 99f
  volar fracture of, 125
  volar tilt of, 118, 118f
Rolando fracture, 150
Ruptured disc, 54

Sacrum
  anteroposterior view of, 38f, 174f, 186f
  lateral view of, 39f, 187f
Sarcroiliac joint, anteroposterior view of, 174f
Scaphoid
  anteroposterior view of, 114f, 140f
  carpal fracture and, 113
  dislocation of, 132, 133f
  fracture of, 126–128, 126f, 127f
  lateral view of, 115f, 141f
  oblique view of, 116f, 141f
Scapholunate joint, 118, 119f
  angle of, 118, 119f
  cortical ring sign of, 133f
  dissociation of, 132
  swelling of, 132
Scapula
  anteroposterior view of, 58f
  axillary view of, 59f
  fracture of, 64, 65f
  tangential "Y" view of, 60f
  transthroacic view of, 61f
Schaphoid
  anteroposterior view of, 126f
  navicular fracture of, 127f
  oblique view of, 127f
  rotary subluxation of, 132, 133f
Seizure, shoulder dislocation and, 72
Sesamoid
  anteroposterior view of, 140f, 258f
  lateral view of, 141f, 259f
  oblique view of, 141f, 260f
Shenton's line
  anteroposterior view of, 186f
  lateral view of, 185, 188f
Shoulder
  acromioclavicular dislocation of, 66, 67f
  anteroposterior view of, 58f, 59f
  axillary view of, 59f
  external rotation of, 69
  forced abduction of, 69
  fracture dislocation of, 74, 75f
  separation of, 66, 67f
  tangential "Y" view of, 60f
  transthoracic view of, 61f
Smith's fracture, 122, 123f
Soft tissue injury, about the knee, 228–230
Spica cast, 128
Spine
  cervical
    anterior dislocation of, 30
    anterior subluxation of, 15, 15f
    anteroposterior view of, 11–12, 12f
    atlanto-axial (C1-C2) instability of, 30, 31f
    "burst" fracture of, 24, 25f
    "clay-shoveler's," 26, 27f
    dislocation of, 12, 32, 33f
    hangman fracture of, 22, 23f
    horizontal translation of, 15f
    injuries of, 11
    instability of, 17, 17f
    Jefferson fracture of, 18, 19f
    lateral relationships of, 16f
    lateral view of, 12, 13f, 15
    lower
      dislocation of, 32, 33f
      subluxation of, 32
    oblique view of, 12, 14f

Spine *(Continued)*
occipital-atlanto (C1) instability of, 28, 29f
odontoid fracture of, 20–21, 21f
open-mouth view of, 12, 13f, 17
posterior dislocation of, 30
rotatory subluxation of, 30
strain on, 34
subluxation of, 32
teardrop fracture of, 24, 25f
lumbar
anteroposterior view of, 38, 38f, 174f
chance fracture of, 50, 51f
herniated nucleus pulposus of, 54
lateral view of, 38, 39f, 40f
oblique view of, 40f
ruptured disc of, 54
spondylolisthesis of, 52, 53f
"spot" lateral view of, 38, 41f
strain of, 54
transverse process fracture of, 48, 49f
wedge fracture of, 46, 47f
lumbosacral, strain of, 54
thoracolumbar
anterioposterior view of, 35, 36f, 37f
chance fracture of, 50, 51f
compression fracture of, 44, 45f
"coned-down" view of, 35
dislocation of, 35
fracture dislocation of, 42, 43f
lateral view of, 37f, 38, 39f, 40f
spondylolisthesis of, 52, 53f
"spot" lateral view of, 38, 41f
transverse process fracture of, 48, 49f
wedge fracture of, 46, 47f
Spinous process
anteroposterior view of, 38f
lateral view of, 39f
oblique view of, 14f
Spondylolisthesis, 52, 53f
Sprain, ankle, 241
Sternoclavicular dislocation, 68
Strap, figure-of-eight, for clavicle fracture, 62
Stress fracture, of metatarsal, 268, 269f
Subtalar joint, dislocation of, 252, 253f
Subtrochanteric fracture, 198
Supracondylar fracture, of humerus, 88, 89f
Surgery, in chronic isthemic spondylolithesis, 52
Symphysis pubis
anteroposterior view of, 186f
lateral view of, 187f
Syndesmosis tear, 246

Talus
anteroposterior view of, 239f, 258f
compression of, 251
dislocation of, 252
fractures of, 252, 253f
lateral view of, 239f, 259f
oblique view of, 260f
subtalar dislocation of, 252, 253f
Tarsometatarsal joint, dislocation of, 264, 265f
Teardrop fracture, of cervical spine, 24, 25f
Terry-Thomas sign, 133f
Thoracolumbar spine
anterioposterior view of, 38, 38f
chance fracture of, 50, 51f
compression fracture of, 44, 45f
"coned-down" view of, 35
fracture dislocation of, 42, 43f
lateral view of, 37f, 38, 39f, 40f
oblique view of, 40f
spondylolisthesis of, 52, 53f
"spot" lateral view of, 38, 41f
transverse process fracture of, 48, 49f
wedge fracture of, 46, 47f
Thumb
anteroposterior view of, 114f
Bennett's fracture dislocation of, 148, 149f
extra-articular fracture of, 151, 151f
Gamekeeper's, 152, 153f
lateral view of, 115f
oblique view of, 116f
Rolando fracture of, 150
spica cast for, 128
"T" fracture of, 150
"Y" fracture of, 150
Tibia
anteroposterior view of, 205f, 221f, 232f, 239f
bicondylar fracture of
anteroposterior view of, 222f
lateral view of, 223f

complex fracture of, 222f, 223f
fracture of, 231–234, 234f, 235f
lateral view of, 206f, 233f, 239f
plateau of, fracture of, 220, 221f–223f
shaft of, anteroposterior view of, 221f–223f
Toe, *see* Metatarsis
Transverse process
anteroposterior view of, 38f
fracture of, 48, 49f
lateral view of, 39f
Trapezium
anteroposterior view of, 114f, 140f
lateral view of, 115f, 141f
oblique view of, 116f, 141f
Trapezoid
anteroposterior view of, 114f, 140f
lateral view of, 115f, 141f
oblique view of, 116f, 141f
Trimalleolar fracture dislocation, 248, 249f
Triquetrum
anteroposterior view of, 114f, 140f
fracture of, 131f
lateral view of, 115f, 141f
oblique view of, 116f, 141f
Trochlea, fracture of, 86

Ulna
coronoid process of, 85f
fracture of
nightstick, 108, 109f
and radius, 106, 107f
Monteggia fracture of, 104, 105f
nightstick fracture of, 108, 109f
olecranon process of, 84f
styloid of
anteroposterior view of, 114f
lateral view of, 115f
oblique view of, 116f
Ulna boot, 241

Vertebra
instability of, 17, 17f
subluxation of, 15, 15f
Volar avulsion fracture, 158, 158f

Wedge fracture, of throacolumbar spine, 46, 47f
"Whiplash," 34
Wrist
anatomic relationships of, 118, 118f, 119f
anteroposterior view of, 114f
Barton's fracture of, 124, 125f
Colle's fracture of, 120, 121f
carpal tunnel view of, 117f
check list, of normal anatomic relationships, 118, 118f, 119f
fracture of, radial head fracture and, 92
hyperextension of, 130
lateral view of, 115f
oblique view of, 116f
Smith's fracture of, 122, 123f
"silver fork" deformity of, 120, 127
volar tilt of, 118, 118f
Wrist drop, 80